The Mercury in Your Mouth

The Mercury in Your Mouth

The Truth About
"Silver" Dental Fillings

Quicksilver Associates

Quicksilver Press
New York, NY

The medical and dental information and procedures in this book are not intended as a substitute for consulting your physician or dentist. They are described here for reference information only. All matters regarding your physical health should be supervised by a qualified medical professional.

Typesetting by Bonnie Freid
Silver card stock from Semper Paper, Union, New Jersey
Cover Designer: Marietta Anastassatos

Library of Congress Catalog # 95-067129
ISBN 0-9643870-0-X

Published by:

Quicksilver Press
211 West 92nd Street, Suite 71
New York, NY 10025
(800) 423-6722
(212) 579-3224

Printed in the United States of America.

10 9 8 7 6 5 4 3 2

In memory of Dr. Linus Pauling,
a wise, brilliant, and courageous scientist,
a kind and compassionate human being.
In honor of one of Pauling's most distinguished
medical disciples, Warren Levin, M.D.
and his wife Susan Levin.

Contents

Symptoms of Mercury Toxicity,   ix

Acknowledgments,   xi

Introduction,   xv

Part One: The Trouble With "Silver" Dental Fillings

1. *They Aren't Really Silver*: Amalgam Dental Fillings and Mercury Toxicity   3

2. What We Know About Mercury   17

Part Two: The Scientific Research

3. The Lorscheider-Vimy Experiments   37

4. The Link Between Mercury and Alzheimer's Disease   53

5. The Immune System, Antibiotic Resistance, and Other Mercury-Linked Syndromes   65

6. Medical Implications of Mercury Toxicity: Alfred A. Zamm, M.D., F.A.C.P.   75

7. The Huggins Diagnostic Center: Hal A. Huggins, D.D.S.   81

Part Three: Mercury and Your Health

8. How Can I Tell If I'm Mercury Toxic?,   87

9. Having Your Fillings Replaced, 113
   (CAUTION: DO NOT DO ANYTHING ABOUT
   HAVING YOUR "SILVER" FILLINGS RE-
   PLACED UNTIL YOU HAVE READ THIS CHAP-
   TER.)

10. Detoxification   123

11. Implications for the Future 131

Appendices

A. Dentists Knowledgeable About Safe Removal of
   Mercury Amalgam "Silver" Fillings 135

B. -Physicians Knowledgeable About the Treat
   ment of Dental-Filling Mercury Toxicity 141

C. General Reading List on Dental Mercury Toxicity
   143

D. Dental Amalgam Mercury, by Fritz L.
   Lorscheider, Ph.D. and Murray Vimy, D.D.S. 147

E. Bibliography of Selected Scientific Research on
   Mercury   153

F. News Clippings   163
   a. German report
   b. San Jose Mercury News
   C. Townsend Letter for Doctors

   Notes   167
   General Index   181
   Index of Proper Names   183

THE FOLLOWING ARE EARLY SYMPTOMS OF MERCURY TOXICITY IF YOU HAVE "SILVER" DENTAL FILLINGS:

Neurological symptoms (from mercury's interference with the nervous system):

- Depression
- Dizziness
- Headaches
- Irritability
- Lack of concentration
- Memory lapses (mild or otherwise)
- Nervousness

Physiological symptoms (from mercury's interference with the immune system, the metabolism, various organs, etc.):

- Allergies
- Bleeding or receding gums (gingivitis)
- Fatigue
- Gastrointestinal illnesses
- High blood pressure
- Kidney problems

Acknowledgments

The true heroes of this book are the scientists who have done the basic research on dental mercury amalgam and its relationship to human illness, along with the small group of dentists and doctors who recognized early on that amalgam fillings are toxic. These men and women were willing to risk criticism, censure, and in the case of clinicians, the potential loss of their licenses, in order to protect their patients' health.

We are deeply grateful to the scientists whose research forms the backbone of this book: Murray Vimy, D.M.D., and Fritz Lorscheider, Ph.D., of the University of Calgary Medical School, Calgary, Alberta; Boyd Haley, Ph.D., of the Lucille Markey Cancer Center, the University of Kentucky; Anne O. Summers, Ph.D., of the University of Georgia; William Markesbery, M.D. and William Ehmann, M.D. of the Sanders Brown Medical Center, University of Kentucky; Vasken Aposhian, Ph.D. and Mary Aposhian, Ph. D., of the University of Arizona School of Pharmacology; and David Eggleston, D.D.S., of the

University of Southern California School of Dentistry.

We wish also to acknowledge the tremendous professional contribution to American dentistry of Hal A. Huggins, D.D.S., of the Huggins Diagnostic Center, Colorado Springs, Colorado. Dr. Huggins was perhaps the first American dentist to recognize the toxicity of amalgam; he deserves much credit for his courage and persistence.

Similarly, Dr. Olympio Pinto of Rio de Janeiro, Brazil may have been the first dentist to give wide publicity to this issue in his own professional practice. He played a large role in spreading the word to Dr. Huggins and many other colleagues in medicine and dentistry.

Special thanks go to Alfred A. Zamm, M.D., of Kingston, New York, who has pioneered in his private practice the treatment of patients suffering from amalgam-induced illness.

We are also indebted to Warren Levin, M.D. and to Mark Breiner, D.D.S., for their wisdom and great professional skill; and to Marty Edelston, founder of Boardroom Reports, who ran several early stories about this issue.

We are grateful to the *FASEB Journal* and to Sandra Jacobson, Executive Editor, for their permission to reprint material from scientific articles first published in their pages, particularly the research of Drs. Lorscheider and Vimy.

The support of G. Tyson Meroon III was crucial to this book's completion.

Finally, we wish to express our sincerest appreciation to Michael Ziff, D.D.S., Executive Director of the International Academy of Oral Medicine and Toxicology, and to Sam Ziff of Bio-Probe, Inc., Orlando, Florida., for their permission to reprint this book a few of the outstanding research reports and charts that were first printed in their publications.

The debt of gratitude that all Americans present and future owe to these dedicated men and women is large indeed.

Quicksilver Associates
211 W. 92nd St., Suite 71
New York, NY 10025

INTRODUCTION: Your "Silver" Dental Fillings Are Toxic

Chronic mercury toxicity from "silver" mercury amalgam dental fillings is the most important unrecognized public health problem of our time. In the 1990's it has just begun to attract public attention, after many years of being invisible to all except the most sophisticated researchers.

It is never easy to acknowledge that a substance which has been thought safe for human use is really unsafe. Dental amalgam has been so widely used for so long ---- since 1833 in the U.S.----that it has been particularly hard to recognize the damage it does to human health. Only when the results of laboratory research reached a critical mass in the 1980s did some of the barriers to public understanding begin to fall.

During the 1990's major scientific and legal advances have been made that signal the end of mercury's use in dentistry. Simultaneously we are beginning a long period of assessing the damage dental amalgam has done to human health, and exploring ways to repair that damage. Some of these developments are:

- On December 16, 1990, 60 MINUTES aired a program on dental mercury amalgam which brought the issue forcefully to public attention. Representatives of organized dentistry subsequently objected strongly to the airing of this program and harshly criticized its production staff, but the program attracted wide media attention and public interest, nevertheless.

- In 1992, Germany banned the use of certain forms of amalgam. The following year, the largest German manufacturer of amalgam, De Gussa, announced that it was voluntarily discontinuing the manufacture of amalgam, partly in order to avoid lawsuits.[1]

- In December 1992, the American Medical Association passed a resolution advocating the elimination of mercury, lead and benzene from all household products, citing their harmful effect on the environment and on human health. [2]

- In August 1995, a Federal court ruled that California's Proposition 65 is valid with regards to dental amalgam, in response to a suit filed by amalgam manufacturers and opposed by San Francisco's Environmental Law Foundation. This means that any dentist who has 10 or more employees must provide "clear and reasonable warning" to both employees and patients that amalgam is a potentially harmful substance.

- In February 1994, the Swedish parliament passed a bill banning all use of dental amalgam by 1997.

The Swedish decision was reached partly on the basis of research carried out at the Carolinska Institut, one of the most prestigious research institutions in the world.4

- On July 11, 1994, the BBC aired a 40-minute documentary on dental amalgam called "The Poison In Your Mouth." It consisted of interviews with prominent scientists involved in research on amalgam toxicity and with officials of the British Dental Association who seemingly were unaware of any research of this kind. The program was shown on the continent July 18 and has since been seen in countries all over the world----all of the the Commonwealth countries except Canada and many others. It has not yet been shown in the U.S. or Canada, allegedly because of pressure from the dental associations and from amalgam manufacturers.

- In early 1995, a legal brief was discovered by documentary film maker John Woods that had been filed by the ADA in a civil lawsuit in Santa Clara, California. The plaintiff, William Tolhurst, D.C., asserted that his amalgam fillings had damaged his health. In this document, attorneys for the ADA argued that

> **The ADA owes no legal duty of care to protect the public from allegedly dangerous products used by dentists. The ADA did not manufacture, design, supply or install the mercury-containing amalgams. The ADA does not control those who do. The ADA's only alleged involvement in the product was to provide information**

regarding its use. Dissemination of information relating to the practice of dentistry does not create a duty of care to protect the public from potential injury." [5]

The American Dental Association thus appears to deny any responsibility for the safety of the general public when the public seeks and receives dental care; and from any responsibility for the competence and knowledge of the ADA's membership in providing that care. Although the Court agreed in this case, it is questionable whether the ADA can maintain such a position permanently and still keep its role as the chief professional organization for dentists.

This statement seems to be a sign that the ADA understands and acknowledges the toxicity of mercury amalgam as a dental filling material and is taking steps to distance itself from liability issues before this toxicity becomes widely known.

For all of these reasons, members of the public need to be informed about the unsafety of dental amalgam, and about how amalgam fillings can be safely removed without further exposing the patient to more mercury vapor.

Practicing dentists should be aware that they have been inadequately informed about amalgam's toxic properties by their professional association, which asserts that it is only a trade association, and that mercury amalgam is safe. Dentists should also know that the ADA has disavowed any duty of care and that individual dentists may therefore be liable to lawsuit in the event of amalgam-caused injury to patients.

We need to know a great deal more about amalgam-related illnesses, how to treat them, and how best to go about detoxification----the removal of mercury stored in body tissues.

In future editions of this book we will include information from readers----physicians, dentists, researchers, and lay persons----who are willing to share their own experiences. We are eager to hear from readers, and we encourage you to write us about treatments that were useful to you.

We would also like to be able to list (with their permission) the names of dentists who understand how to remove mercury fillings with proper protection for the patient, and of physicians who have successfully treated mercury-toxic patients. If you know a dentist or physician in these categories who is willing to be listed in future editions of this book, please let us know.

PART ONE

The Trouble With "Silver" Dental Fillings

CHAPTER 1

They Aren't Really Silver: Amalgam Dental Fillings and Mercury Toxicity

In the ordinary course of live, approximately 95% of the adult population of the United States is exposed to mercury every day. What this means for the individual is that most Americans are in constant contact with one of the most toxic metals in existence, without realizing it.

Mercury is much more toxic than arsenic or cadmium It is more toxic than lead, whose presence in the human environment has become an object of great public concern over the past fifteen years. The maximum amount of mercury that the Environmental Protection Agency allows people to be exposed to is 5,000 times smaller than the permissible amount of lead exposure; in other words, the EPA apparently considers mercury to be 5,000 times more toxic than lead.[6] The only metals that are more poisonous than mercury are osmium and the radioactive metals such as plutonium, radium and polonium.

The mercury that you absorb finds its way to your

brain, heart, liver, gastrointestinal tract, endocrine glands, kidneys and muscles. In the body mercury is stored in tissue, and it is released extremely slowly, at varying rates of speed from different types of tissue.

Very few of us are aware of this continuing toxic exposure. Partly this is because our contact with mercury is internal: the mercury is inside our bodies, and we inhale and swallow substantial amounts without realizing it.

But the main reason for our lack of awareness is that our mercury exposure is not presented to us for what it is. There is a simple and unexpected source for the mercury that we are exposed to: ordinary "silver" dental fillings.

The longstanding use of the term "silver dental fillings" gives the impression that these fillings are really made of silver—that beautiful precious metal from which the most valuable tableware is fashioned. But although their name and appearance suggest that the fillings are made of silver, they are not. They are composed of "amalgam"—by definition an alloy of mercury with other metals.

It is mercury which forms the highest percentage of this alloy.

Contemporary amalgam is approximately **50% mercury by weight;** older fillings often had a higher percentage of mercury, between 55% and 75%. The remainder of the filling is made up of other metals, such as silver, copper, zinc and tin.

The second term used for these fillings—"amalgam"Ñis equally unclear because it is not widely recognizable to the public as a substance that contains mercury. Because these common terms lend themselves to misinterpretation, "mercury amalgam" will be used in this book.

Dental fillings are small, but the amount of mercury in a filling is not inconsequential. A standard physician's thermometer contains 700 mg. of mercury sealed in glass. A large mercury amalgam filling contains more—an average of 750 mg. mercury,[7] with one or more surfaces completely exposed to the air and to any food or drink that you put in your mouth.

Bridges and root canals packed with amalgam can contain much larger quantities.

In short, the trouble with "silver" dental fillings is that they're not really made of silver, but of mercury. And mercury is a poison.

IS THE MERCURY
IN DENTAL FILLINGS STABLE?

Ever since the use of mercury amalgam in dentistry was introduced into the United States from France by the Crawcour brothers in 1833[8], dentists who favored its use have asserted that once mercury amalgam has "set" it is stable. In other words, once a filling has hardened after being placed in a tooth, no mercury would escape from it. For many years there was no scientific method available for testing this contention one way or the other.

In the early 1980's, a research group headed by two scientists at the University of Calgary Medical School—Dr. Murray Vimy, D.M.D. (a practicing dentist in Calgary who is on the Medical School faculty) and Dr. Fritz Lorscheider (an American who is Professor of Medical Physiology at Calgary)—began using newly available, sophisticated analytical instruments to examine the behavior of the mercury in amalgam fillings. Several other research groups which preceded them had produced good scientific work which indicated that amalgam fillings might indeed be toxic; Lorscheider and Vimy decided to try to settle the matter once and for all.

Vimy and Lorscheider's research produced startling and disturbing results. Their team demonstrated conclusively that mercury amalgam is not stable at all. **Mercury vapor is continuously released from amalgam fillings in measurable quantities, from the moment the fillings are inserted into your teeth.** This mercury vapor is inhaled and swallowed, and is absorbed into every part of your body.

This instability of dental mercury amalgam has been confirmed by other scientists working independently. For example, Dr. James V. Masi, an engineer at Western New England College in Springfield, Massachusetts who is a specialist in metals corrosion, has shown that amalgam fillings are self-corroding because of the mixture of metals, and that different "qualities" of amalgam can corrode each other, releasing mercury vapor into the mouth air.

In short, if you have "silver" fillings, every time you take a breath, you inhale a little bit of one of the most poisonous substances on earth—mercury vapor. And while the body can cope to some extent with small amounts of poisons, too much exposure can cause its coping ability to break down.

The research generated by Lorscheider, Vimy and their colleagues is so carefully constructed and performed that it has established as scientific fact the instability of mercury amalgam dental fillings. The reports of their experiments have been published in the most highly respected and most stringently peer-reviewed scientific journals.

The presence of this powerful poison inside the body has far-reaching and serious implications. Studies done on mercury toxicity—especially on incidents where a number of people were exposed to mercury in industrial accidents or in the use of mercury-treated seed grain for food[9]—link it with a number of illnesses. These include allergies; chronic fatigue; depression; gastrointestinal tract disorders; gingivitis (another name for periodontal disease, i.e., bleeding gums); immune system weakness; neurological problems; reproductive and fertility disorders; birth defects, especially damage to the fetus' nervous system; kidney disease, heart problems, hypertension, antibiotic resistance, respiratory tract disorders, hearing and vision difficulties, and skin disorders such as dermatitis and eczema.

This may sound like a long collection of problems to be generated by one element. In fact, it is a highly selective list, designed to give you a concise idea of the wide range of physical symptoms which can be associated with mercury amalgam fillings.

Poisons and toxins absorbed in small amounts over a long period of time affect individuals very differently because of the principle of *biological individuality*. Each individual is biologically different from every other, and as a result each body's reactions and responses will be different.

The genetic "weak link" in your physical makeup is the area where a problem is likely to arise first if you are exposed to mercury. One person may develop irritable bowel syndrome or some other type of gastrointestinal tract disorder. Another may be vulnerable in the respiratory tract and develop severe asthma or bronchitis. A third may experience hearing loss and dizziness but have no other signs of illness. A fourth may be troubled by an unexplained loss of energy and physical clumsiness. A fifth may have memory problems; and so on.

A chart showing symptoms relieved following the removal of amalgam fillings gives a stunning idea of the extent of mercury's possible involvement in health problems throughout our population. A "Consolidated Symptom Analysis of 1569 Patients" was published in the March 1993 issue of **Bio-Probe**, a newsletter published by Orlando, Florida publisher Sam Ziff and his son, Michael Ziff, D.D.S.

The Ziffs took a series of studies and reports examining the adverse effects of mercury, and combined them in a single symptom list. These included 762 Patient Adverse Reaction Reports submitted to the FDA by patients who had had their amalgams replaced. The reports **"reflect the individual's assessment of any changes that may have occurred in their health status as a direct result."**[10]

In addition, the Ziffs included 519 patients from Sweden, reported by Mats Hanson, Ph.D., a Swedish mercury researcher; 100 patients from Denmark studied by Henrik Lichtenberg, D.D.S.; 80 patients from Canada reported by Pierre Larose, D.D.S.: 86 patients from Colorado, reported by Robert L. Siblerud, O.D., M.S.; and 22 patients reported by Alfred V. Zamm, M.D., FACI, FACP, of Kingston, New York.

As one example of the symptoms relieved, let's take the first item, allergies. 14.5% of the group reported allergies. **89% of these allergy sufferers reported improvement or cure after amalgam fillings were replaced.**

Table 1.1 Selected Health Symptom Analysis of 1569 Patients Who Eliminated Mercury-Containing Dental Fillings.

The following represents a partial statistical symptom summary of 1569 patients who participated in six different studies evaluating the health effects of replacing mercury-containing dental fillings with non-mercury containing dental fillings. The data was derived from the following studies: 762 Patient Adverse Reaction Reports submitted to the FDA by the individual patients; 519 patients in Sweden reported on by Mats Hanson, Ph.D.; 100 patients in Denmark performed by Henrik Lichtenberg, D.D.S.; 80 patients in Canada performed by Pierre Larose, D.D.S.; 86 patients in Colorado reported on by Robert L. Siblerud, O.D., M.S., as partial fulfillment of a Ph.D. requirement and 22 patients reported on by Alfred V. Zamm, M.D., FACA, FACP. The combined total of all patients participating in the six studies was 1569.

% of Total Reporting	Symptom	Number Reporting	Number Improved or Cured	% of Cure or Improvement
14%	Allergy	221	196	89%
5%	Anxiety	86	80	93%
5%	Bad temper	81	68	89%
6%	Bloating	88	70	88%
6%	Blood pressure problems	99	53	54%
5%	Chest pains	79	69	87%
22%	Depression	347	315	91%
22%	Dizziness	343	301	88%
45%	Fatigue	705	603	86%
15%	Gastrointestinal problems	231	192	83%
8%	Gum problems	129	121	94%
34%	Headaches	531	460	87%
3%	Migraine headaches	45	39	87%
12%	Insomnia	187	146	78%
10%	Irregular heartbeat	159	139	87%
8%	Irritability	132	119	90%
17%	Lack of concentration	270	216	80%
6%	Lack of energy	91	88	97%

% of Total Reporting	Symptom	Number Reporting	Number Improved or Cured	% of Cure or Improvement
17%	Memory loss	265	193	73%
17%	Metallic taste	260	247	95%
7%	Multiple sclerosis	113	86	76%
8%	Muscle tremor	126	104	83%
10%	Nervousness	158	131	83%
8%	Numbness anywhere	118	97	82%
20%	Skin disturbances	310	251	81%
9%	Sore throat	149	128	86%
6%	Tachycardia	97	68	70%
4%	Thyroid problems	56	44	79%
12%	Ulcers & sores in oral cavity	189	162	86%
7%	Urinary tract problems	115	87	76%
29%	Vision problems	462	289	63%

Anyone who has serious allergies knows how miraculous it would be to have one's symptoms improve significantly or, better yet, disappear. Billions of dollars are spent in the U.S. every year on allergy relief in a variety of forms. If there were a new treatment for allergies whose research background showed that 89% of everyone who tried it got a lot better or was cured, it would be hailed as a major scientific breakthrough.

Well—here it is! But it involves taking a toxic substance *out of* the body, rather than putting a medication *into it*.

The percentage of allergy sufferers in this collection of reports was relatively small. Much larger percentages of respondents reported suffering from fatigue (45%); headaches (34%); depression (22%); and dizziness (22%). **86% of the fatigue sufferers, 87% of the headache victims, 91% of those with depression and 88% of those with dizziness reported cure or improvement after the removal of their amalgam fillings.**

The Ziffs remarked that this relief of allergies would not be expected from reading a report published in January 1993 by the U.S. Public Health Service. The Committee to Coordinate Environmental Health and Related Programs was asked to prepare a report on the potential toxicity of dental amalgam. Concerning allergies, it wrote:

> **"Only a small proportion of mercury-sensitized individuals respond adversely to the placement of amalgam restorations. The few case reports of adverse allergic reactions to amalgam involve skin reactions, such as rashes and eczematous lesions...**[11]

The Ziffs point out that this statement completely ignores

> **valid peer-reviewed scientific studies demonstrating an allergic reaction to dental amalgam ranging from 16.5% for non-allergic patients to 44% for fourth year dental students. More importantly, as this symptom analysis demonstrates, the question is not whether the patient is allergic to dental amalgam but rather the direct causal relationship of mercury/amalgam dental fillings to the development of allergies to food, chemicals, and environmental factors. In our analysis, this is supported by the fact that 14% of the individuals reported some type**

**of allergy and that after replacement of their
mercury/amalgam dental fillings, 89% of the
group reported their condition had improved or
was totally eliminated.**

**If you were to extrapolate this data to the ap-
proximately 140 million amalgam bearers in the
United States, there should be 19.5 million people (14%) with amalgam causally related allergies. Of this number 89% or approximately 17.4
million would have their allergies ameliorate or
disappear simply by having their mercury dental fillings exchanged for non-mercury ones.**[12]

The highest incidence of improvement was for the
small percentage (6%) reporting lack of energy. **97%
of these reported cure or improvement.**

The two lowest incidences of improvement were
just **54% improvement for the 6% who reported
blood pressure problems;** and **63% for the 29%
who had vision problems**—a condition that few
physicians would even dream of ascribing to dental
fillings.

In other words, **in the lowest-improved groups,
over half the complaint group experienced cure
or improvement. For all the other complaint
groups, the rate of improvement was between 70
and 97%, including a stunning 75% improvement
for the 7% suffering from Multiple Sclerosis.**

This statistic is perhaps the most astonishing in
the entire group, since traditional medicine would be
most unlikely under any circumstances to consider
that there might be a connection between MS and the
composition of the patient's dental fillings.

These are, quite simply, extraordinary results.
There are very few treatments of any kind for physical illness which yield such high improvement rates.

Only antibiotics (before the development of antibiotic resistance) and some vaccines—like the Salk polio vaccine—have effectiveness rates that are as high or higher. Moreover, because these results come from such a wide collection of different groups, crossing national and geographical boundaries, they seem to have broad application.

But we should also note that in one respect, these figures drawn from patient reports could be conservative. The researchers did not take into account the fact that the mercury used in fillings tends to be eliminated from the body very slowly, over a period of years rather than months or weeks. If the individuals surveyed had been questioned again five years later, larger percentages of respondents might have reported cures and improvement.

There is a biochemical reason for this huge variety of symptoms. Mercury is a *cytotoxin:* it is poisonous to all living cells. It also has the capacity to bond with any chemical which contains a particular type of molecule called a "sulfhydryl," found in most proteins. The human body contains an enormous number of protein compounds; they are the building blocks for all body tissue, and many have one or more sulfhydryl groups.

As a result, mercury can interfere with virtually any process or organ in the body. It can combine with a protein in the skin and cause skin disorders such as dermatitis; it can accumulate in the nervous system and cause a wide variety of nervous system disorders, manifested as physical or emotional illness. The expression "mad as a hatter" comes from a time when hatters processed their own felt using mercury and became deranged from inhaling mercury vapor.

There are other physical illnesses which can now be identified as related in some way to the mercury syndrome.

Mercury accumulation in the brain from dental-filling amalgam is suspected of being one primary cause of Alzheimer's Disease.

Research on this subject has been under way for several years, carried out by two different scientific teams at the University of Kentucky, one led by Dr. William Markesbery, Director of the Sanders Brown Center on Aging, and Dr.William Ehmann and one by Dr. Boyd Haley of the Lucille Markey Cancer Center. In addition, Drs. Fritz Lorscheider and Murray Vimy are also engaged in studies related to amalgam and Alzheimer's.

Mercury also has a marked negative effect on the immune system.

A preliminary study conducted by a Los Angeles dentist, Dr. David W. Eggleston, indicated that **the presence of mercury amalgam dental fillings in the mouth reduces the efficiency of the immune system by one-third to one-half.**[13] This is research which should be expanded and carried farther and whose results should be widely available to the public, particularly to those whose immune system is compromised. It is especially important for those who are HIV positive and for people battling illnesses such as cancer.

The message is very plain: if your health is a problem in some respect and you have "silver" fillings in your teeth, the most recent research suggests that the presence of these fillings may be a contributing or primary cause of your physical illnesses. In a nation increasingly concerned about the rising cost of health care, dental amalgam may be an unsuspected factor which causes or intensifies any number of physical illnesses—and which multiplies health care costs many times over.

The first two chapters of this book give an introduction to this problem. Next come a series of chapters that outline the development of contemporary scientific research on mercury amalgam. The third section of the book details the physical impact of mercury toxicity, and how to identify its symptoms. Also included is a chapter on various detoxification methods that are in the process of development.

Finally, there are appendices of scientific and other references, including a brief list of some of the dentists and physicians who have experience with filling replacement and mercury toxicity problems.

SUMMARY -They Aren't Really Silver

1. "Silver" dental fillings are not made chiefly of silver. They are made of an alloy called amalgam whose principal ingredient is mercury, a highly toxic heavy metal. New contemporary fillings contain about 50% mercury by weight; older fillings were made of formulas contained as much as 75% mercury.

Reliable scientific research shows that:

2. If you have "silver" dental fillings, you have absorbed mercury from them continuously since they were inserted. As a result you have mercury in your body tissues.

3. You will continue to absorb mercury from these mercury amalgam fillings as long as you have

them in your teeth, and you will gradually accumulate higher and higher levels of mercury.

4. The degree to which your "mercury body burden"
    affects your health depends on several factors:

    • The number, size, and mercury content of your
       fillings. How many do you have? Are they large
       or small? Are they recent fillings—50% mer-
       cury—or old fillings whose original percentage
       of mercury was higher?

    • Your body mass. Are you tall or short, slender
       or stout? If you are 5'1" and weigh 100 pounds,
       you may be affected more strongly by your
       fillings than a person who is, say, 6'2" tall and
       weighs 200 pounds. Children can be affected
       particularly strongly by amalgam fillings be-
       cause their body mass is so small.

    • How sensitive you are to mercury. Individuals
       differ in their sensitivity even to a toxic sub-
       stance like mercury. This doesn't mean that
       less-sensitive people aren't affected by expo-
       sure to mercury; it means that they just take
       longer to show symptoms. We will discuss in a
       later chapter how your degree of mercury sen-
       sitivity can be tested.

5. If you have chronic health problems for which
    you have been unable to find a cause or a cure
    and you have "silver" mercury fillings, you may
    be suffering from some degree of mercury toxic-
    ity.

CHAPTER 2

What We Know About Mercury

The information contained in this book is based on research designed and carried out by scientists—physicians, physiologists, pathologists, toxicologists, biochemists, molecular biologists and dentists. Reports of their research have been published in scientific journals, after being subjected to strict peer review by other experts in their fields. Several scientific bibliographies, along with a list of books for the general reader, are included at the end of this book for those who wish to read more.

Most people are surprised to learn that there is a large body of well-designed, well-respected research documenting the negative effect of mercury—including dental-filling mercury—on both animal and human health. Some of these studies date back as far as the 1930's, a period in which a great deal of important biochemical research was done (Vitamin C and several of the B-complex vitamins, for example, were discovered and named in the 1930's).

WHAT IS MERCURY?

Mercury is a metal, numbered 80 on the periodic table of elements. It is a silvery liquid at room temperature, a property that is unique among metals. It is also unstable, emitting mercury vapor from the surface of its liquid droplets at ordinary room temperatures. It is the second most poisonous metal known to exist.[14]

Mercury was known and its properties recognized as far back as classical Greek civilization. Aristotle named it "living silver" or "quicksilver" because of its extremely fast reaction to an outside stimulus. Its scientific symbol "Hg" stands for the Greek name *Hydrargentum*, "water silver." At room temperature, liquid elemental mercury is extremely volatile, responding with lightening swiftness to the slightest movement or touch.

Mercury's responsiveness made it a standard ingredient in thermometers because it would expand quickly in reaction to a change in heat or cold, rising within a narrow tube to a level which could be exactly measured to tell the temperature. Its strong electrical properties make it a standard ingredient in batteries. Mercury has a negative valence and easily exchanges charged ions with other metals, creating an electrical circuit. An ordinary alkaline AA Everready battery contains a minimal quantity of mercury: .02% mercury by weight, or 4.5 mg.

AN ANCIENT POISON

There has never been any question about mercury's status as a poison. Two thousand five hundred years ago, the ancient Greeks were vividly aware of its poisonous qualities. Mercury was employed as a murder weapon by pouring it into the victim's ear, where it paralyzed the brain and caused almost instantaneous death. Centuries later, in Shakespeare's play, Hamlet's father was dispatched by the identical use of another poison, "henbane," which the dramatist noted was similar to quicksilver in its effects:

> ...And in the porches of my ears did pour
> The leperous distillment, whose effect
> Holds such an enmity with blood of man
> That swift as quicksilver it courses through
> The natural gates and alleys of the body,
> And with a natural vigor it doth posset
> And curd, like eager drippings into milk,
> The thin and wholesome blood. So it did mine.
>
> ----Hamlet, Act 1, Sc.V, ll. 63-70

Lewis Carroll immortalized the effects of mercury for English-speaking civilization in the "Mad Hatter," a character in **ALICE IN WONDERLAND**. The Hatter runs around talking distractedly in incoherent phrases and is unable to concentrate on anything for more than a second or two. This comical creature was based upon a widely recognized phenomenon in the 18th and 19th centuries, when hatters often displayed these symptoms as a result of breathing mercury vapor while they processed hat felt. There was a hat-making center in Connecticut recently enough that victims of Hatter's Disease still live in this area of Connecticut and display the disease's symptoms.

Mercury's toxicity is openly acknowledged in that most American and most accessible source of knowledge, the encyclopedia. Four different encyclopedias,

available in any library and some in many homes
have short but comprehensive descriptions of mercury's effect on living organisms:

From the Encyclopedia Americana:

**Mercury-Vapor Poisoning. Poisoning from
mercury-vapor inhalation has long been an industrial hazard in electrical apparatus manu-
facturing and other industries using large
amounts of mercury. In the body, inhaled mercury vapor is largely oxidized to inorganic mercury, which becomes concentrated in the kidneys and causes an increase in the output of
urine (diuresis). Other early symptoms include
blurred vision, bleeding gums, and a metallic
taste in the mouth. With continued exposure
there may be muscle tremors, loss of appetite,
and emotional disturbance. Often, the symptoms clear up when the person is no longer
exposed to the vapor. [New York: Grolier Limited, 1990. Vol. I8 (M to Mexico City), p. 722.]**

From the Enyclopedia Britannica:

**Chronic mercury poisoning results from expo-
sure to small amounts of mercury over ex-
tended periods of time... The symptoms are
loss of appetite, salivation, gingivitis, nutritional disturbances, increasing renal damage,
and anemia. The treatment consists of removal
of the patient from all contact with mercury or
its compounds, promotion of elimination, and
improvement of the patient's nutritive state.
Response is sometimes very slow. (Chicago,
London, etc., 1967, Vol. 15 (Maximinus to
Naples, Kingdom of, p. 184.)**

From theMcGraw-Hill Encylopedia of Science & Technology:

> Mercury and almost all its compounds are quite poisonous to man and animals. In chronic mercury poisoning, reddening and bleeding of the gums, digestive disturbances, deafness, and tremors of the hands occur. (New York: McGraw-Hill, 1982, p.304.)

From Van Nostrand's Scientific Encyclopedia:

> Toxicity: Mercury and its compounds, with few exceptions, are highly poisonous to living organisms. Mercury can cause acute renal failure and nephrotic syndrome. Chronic exposure to or ingestion of mercury may lead to polyneuropathy. Confirmation of poisoning is sometimes made by analysis for the presence of mercury in hair, fingernails, serum, and urine. Removal of the metal may be hastened by the oral administration several times a day of d-penacillamine. (Sixth Edition, Volume II. Douglas M. Considine, P.E., Editor, and Glenn D. Considine, Managing Editor. New York, Van Nostrand Reinhold Company, 1983, p.1857-58.)

The most widely-respected toxicological manual, Goodman and Gilman's *The Pharmacological Basis of Therapeutics* (Eighth Edition, Pergamon Press, 1990) elaborates on these details considerably.

> Toxicity. *Elemental Mercury.* Short-term exposure to elemental mercury vapor may produce symptoms within several hours; these include weakness, chills, metallic taste, nausea, vomiting, diarrhea, dyspnea, cough, and a feeling

of tightness in the chest. Pulmonary toxicity may progress to an interstitial pneumonitis with severe compromise of respiratory function. Recovery, although usually complete, may be complicated by residual interstitial fibrosis.

Chronic exposure to mercury vapor produces a more insidious form of toxicity that is dominated by neurological effects (Friberg and Vostal, 1972). The syndrome is referred to as the asthenic vegetative syndrome and consists of neurasthenic symptoms in addition to three or more of the following findings (Goyer, 1985): goiter, increased uptake of radioiodine by the thyroid, tachycardia, labile pulse, gingivitis, dermographia, and increased mercury in the urine. With continued exposure, tremor becomes quite noticable and psychological changes consist of depression, irritability, excessive shyness, insomnia, emotional instability, forgetfulness, confusion, and vasomotor disturbances (such as excessive perspiration and uncontrolled blushing, which together are referred to as erethism.) Common features of intoxication from mercury vapor are severe salivation and gingivitis. The triad of increased excitability, tremors, and gingivitis has been recognized historically as the major manifestation of exposure to mercury vapor when mercury nitrate was used in the fur, felt and hat industries. Renal dysfunction has also been reported to result from long-term industrial exposure to mercury vapor. Goodman and Gilman's *The Pharmacological Basis of Therapeutics* (Eighth Edition, Pergamon Press, 1990) pp.1599-1600.

Modern safety standards have regulated very

strictly the amount of mercury workers can be exposed to in a day and the way in which mercury can be handled. Dental office personnel are particularly vulnerable. University of Southern California Dental School faculty member Dr. David Eggleston writes,

Dental amalgam is classified as a hazardous material by the OSHA, and excess dental amalgam must be disposed of according to its Material Safety Data Sheet. If the exact amount of dental amalgam could be mixed for each restoration, all of the amalgam could be placed in the patient's tooth. Invariably, there is excess to be rid of. The ADA recommends the following:

"All amalgam scraps should be salvaged and stored in a tightly closed container. The scrap should be covered by a sulfide solution such as x-ray or photographic fixer solution.
A no-touch technique of handling amalgam should be used. Skin that is exposed to mercury should be cleaned. Precapsulated alloy should be used. Water spray and high-volume evacuation should be used when removing old or finishing new dental restorations. Evacuation systems should be passed through filters, strainers, or traps. A face mask should be used to avoid breathing amalgam dust."

From *Dental Amalgam: A Review of the Literature*, David W. Eggleston, D.D.S.

In 1992, the World Health Organization declared that there is no safe level of mercury for human beings—in other words, mercury is so poisonous that **no amount of mercury absorption is safe.**

However, the body of scientific research on amalgam fillings shows that a person who has amalgam fillings absorbs from 3 to 17 micrograms of mercury daily—**far more than the .03 nanogam level of mercury which the Environmental Protection Agency mandates as the maximum allowable amount for industrial workers!**[15]

It is not just mercury vapor that is released from mercury dental fillings. They also create a phenomenon called "electrogalvinism," or electricity in the mouth. This is the phenomenon which on occasion has caused people to pick up radio stations on their dental fillings, or to experience small electric shocks in the mouth when eating or drinking.

In 1994, Prof. James V. Masi published a paper on "Corrosion of Restorative Materials: The Problem and the Promise." [16] Masi defines corrosion as "the destruction or deterioration of a material because of its interaction with its environment." The type of corrosion that occurs in dental fillings is electro-chemical: the metal with the more positive charge serves as a cathode (the pole which releases electrically charged ions), while the metal with the more negative charge serves as an anode (the point which receives the charged ions and where corrosion takes place).

Pure gold, which has a high positive charge (+0.26) causes a high rate of corrosion of the negatively-charged mercury(-0.16) in amalgam fillings, and its release into the body. Titanium, which has a smaller positive charge (+0.5) than gold, and silver and stainless steel with smaller negative charges (-0.05 and -0.10 respectively) than mercury also cause corrosion and release of mercury from amalgams.

Ultimately, because of the mixture of metals found in dental amalgam, Masi concludes that "amalgams are potentially self-corroding ..., and amalgams of different "quality" corrode each other as well. Regions of stress further enhance the corrosion process and lead to stress corrosion and stress corrosion cracking."

As part of his research, Masi examined over sixty samples of amalgam restorations in their host teeth. He sliced the teeth into sections and analyzed them using standard metallurgical techniques. Three noticeable common factors were found. First, the samples all showed some degree of micro-cracking, regardless of age. Second, mercury migrated from the filling into the material of the tooth so that "mercury levels are detectable at many millimeters from the (filling) margin." Mercury migration was faster along the lines of the micro-cracks.

Finally, Masi found that "mechanical pressure of less than 2000 Pa on the amalgam surface always produced 'droplets' of mercury, exclusive of the age of the restoration." Electron micrograph photos of these phenomena are included in Masi's paper.

MERCURY AS A DENTAL-FILLING MATERIAL

If mercury is so toxic, and if all mercury fillings release mercury vapor and droplets into the body, how did we ever come up with the idea of putting mercury in our mouths in the first place?

The mouth, after all, is not just the opening through which we absorb both solid and liquid food and some air; it is also constantly bathed in saliva, which can be expected to absorb microscopic particles of any substance in the mouth that is not completely inert.

The use of mercury amalgam as a filling material supposedly originated in England around 1825, and was carried to the Continent almost immediately. In 1833 it was brought to the United States by two semi-charlatans named the Crawcour brothers, who inspired suspicion in the more conservative American dentists by their extravagant claims.

Early 19th century dentists had **NO** cheap, effective, and easily workable filling material. Gold was effective, but it was expensive and had to be cast. Silver provided similar obstacles. Lead was soft but had to be heated in order to be installed, and frequently split the tooth when it cooled. Amalgam possessed the perfect combination of properties: it was malleable when the mercury was first mixed with the other metals and then hardened into a durable filling.

When amalgam was introduced into the U.S., there were initially many dentists who believed that it was unsafe because of its mercury content. The huckster-like behavior of the men who brought it to this country did not help that impression. The German word for "quicksilver" was "Quecksilber;" American dentists shortened the word to "quack" to describe the amalgam-hucksters, and the term became part of the English language. It is sobering to realize that the original "quacks" were dentists who advocated the use of mercury amalgam and that most dentists are still advocating it today.

By 1845 the controversy had become vigorous enough to be named "The First Amalgam War," and to split apart the Society of Dental Surgeons, the original professional association for dentists. Ultimately the Society of Dental Surgeons died. The amalgam-oriented dentists formed their own group in 1899, the American Dental Association. American dentists have employed amalgam as their filling material of choice ever since.

It is interesting to note that a suspicion of amalgam endured in the minds of some dentists in New York City, where the original controversy ran high and a trace of its memory remained. There has always been a tiny percentage of New York City dentists who believed that amalgam was dangerous and who gave their patients only gold fillings, telling them that gold was a safer material as well as being more durable.

In addition to its victory in the first dental wars on amalgam, mercury has been a familiar element in the American home for most of us who are now adults. We played with mercury as children, in that innocent age before Americans were aware that substances like lead, asbestos and mercury are toxic. We had mercury antiseptics put on our skinned knees and elbows in the form of merthiolate or merchurochrome. We got mercury-containing calomine lotion daubed on our chicken pox sores to ease the pain and itching. Many women in the past 50 years have used contraceptive gels that contain mercury - mercury is so poisonous that it is a superior sperm-killer. Even some contemporary antihistamine nose sprays (like Afrin) contain .02% of a mercury compound as a preservative—just a tiny bit of the stuff will kill any bacteria around. Our exposure to mercury is not unique to dental fillings. But dental fillings make up by far the largest part of our exposure.

As we have noted before, a standard physician's thermometer contains 700mg of pure mercury.[17] A large dental filling contains 750 mg or more of mercury.[18] If any one of us were to take twelve to twenty thermometers into the main entryway of our house

or apartment, break the thermometer glass, and scat-
ter the mercury around----and then notify the EPA
about what had been done----the EPA could quarantine the house or apartment until the mercury had
been cleaned up.

Yet large numbers of Americans have twelve to
twenty mercury amalgam fillings in their mouths----
and some of those fillings undoubtedly contain more
amalgam than a standard thermometer. The mouth
is a far smaller and more dangerous place for mercury
than your front hall. The mercury vapor that you
inhale into your sinuses and lungs from your fillings
is much more concentrated than any you might inhale in the comparatively large space of an entry hall.

Nevertheless, we think nothing of living for years
with large quantities of mercury inside our mouths,
in our teeth, constantly releasing mercury vapor into
our bodies through a number of different pathways.

As Dr. Michael Ziff once remarked: "You wouldn't
take a leaky thermometer, put it in your mouth, and
leave it there 24 hours a day, 365 days a year. Yet
that's exactly what happens when an amalgam filling
is installed in your mouth."

These examples are not exaggerated. The mercury
in your thermometer is exactly the same mercury that
is used in your "silver" dental fillings. The mercury in
your teeth has exactly the same capacity for damaging
your body as the mercury from your thermometer.

However, there are fewer controls on the mercury
in your mouth than there are on the mercury in your
thermometer or on the floor of your front hall. A
manufacturer who makes a leaky thermometer can
be fined for potentially damaging human health.

The EPA can mandate a quarantine and clean-up

of a mercury spill in your home, because it is a threat to human health.

However, there are no restrictions of any kind against a dentist's placing large or small amounts of mercury in your teeth. The dentist doesn't even have to inform you that the mercury in the filling material is potentially toxic.

Despite the weight of scientific knowledge, the subject of mercury's use for dental fillings in the human mouth remains controversial as far as public dialogue is concerned.

It's true that as a general principle, some caution may be appropriate in making important alterations in medical or dental treatments, because of the enormous disruption that such changes can create.

When mercury amalgam is openly acknowledged to be poisonous and harmful to human beings, major changes will be mandated for the dental profession— a situation which could bring concern and upheaval to American dentistry. Conceivably such a change might adversely affect the quality of care being offered for a period of time.

Many dentists have not received formal education in handling the new composite filling materials, and would have to be retrained to use these more complex restorative substances. Most dentists have been trained to use gold for fillings and crowns—but although gold is the most durable filling material in existence, and is not reactive in the body, it is much more expensive than any other filling material and also more complicated to install. The widespread use of gold would greatly increase the cost of dental fillings.

On the other side of the argument, however, if the toxic effect of the fillings is not disclosed, there are

even more negative implications for the well-being of
the millions of people who have amalgam fillings and
whose health may be at risk now or in the future
because of mercury's powerful toxic impact.

THE SLOW SPREAD OF INFORMATION

The first impulse of many readers of this book will
undoubtedly be to ask their personal dentist about
this research and about how mercury toxicity might
affect them.

There are a few dentists who have been aware of
the hazards of mercury amalgam fillings for a long
time. Brazil's Dr. Olympio Pinto learned about the toxicity of amalgam fillings from his dentist father, and
has been replacing amalgams with non-toxic materials
for decades. Dr. Pinto explained the rationale for his
stance on amalgam to an American dentist, Dr. Hal A.
Huggins of Colorado Springs, Colo. When Huggins
saw patients recover from a variety of conditions after
the removal of their amalgams, he built his practice on
the treatment of mercury toxicity in patients with
amalgams.Over the years many other American dentists learned about amalgam toxicity and also stopped
using dental mercury amalgam.

However, your dentist may know little or nothing
about the the research which shows that mercury
amalgams is toxic.

In the most extreme instances, some dentists may
not know that this research has been done at all.

There is a curious but very simple reason for this.
Scientific research tends to be compartmentalized by
discipline. With a few outstanding exceptions (Drs.
Eggleston, Vimy, and Ziff) most scientific research on
amalgam toxicity has been done by physicians and
Ph.D. scientists, not by dentists. As a result dentists

are generally not familiar with this research. Dentists, medical doctors, and scientific researchers are members of completely separate professions with separate professional associations and information networks. They publish papers on their research in totally different professional journals.

Moreover, the research on dental mercury toxicity has in many cases been carried out by specialized academic researchers who publish in journals mainly read by researchers in their own field. Dr. Fritz Lorscheider, for example, is a fetal physiologist; Dr. Boyd Haley, at the University of Kentucky, is a biochemist; Dr. Anne Summers, at the Univeristy of Georgia, is a molecular biologist. Practicing physicians normally don't read these extremely specialized journals in which such research scientists' reports appear—-such as The FASEB Journal, The Journal of Toxicology, and Brain Research—because they just don't have the time.

In addition to this compartmentalization of scientific, medical and dental research, the American Dental Association has appeared very reluctant to acknowledge that mercury amalgam is toxic and has been slow to communicate to its membership the most recent and alarming evidence about mercury amalgam's role in physical illnesses. As a result, many dentists are unaware of it.

The majority of dentists have been told by their teachers, their colleagues, and their professional association that mercury amalgam is perfectly all right as long as it has hardened. **They genuinely do not know that that information is incorrect and outdated.** So don't be surprised if that is what your dentist tells you.

There is also a potent psychological factor in-

volved. No one in a healing profession likes to dis-
cover that their well-meaning efforts have been
achieving the opposite effect. Dentists go into dentistry for a variety of reasons, but one reason certainly is that dentistry is a healing profession and its
members are highly respected. The natural tendency
for many dentists, therefore, is to wait and see, and
meanwhile not to alarm their patients about possible
toxic effects which their professional association says
don't exist.

YOUR RIGHT TO SELF-DETERMINATION

But your fillings are in *your* mouth—not your dentist's—and whatever symptoms you have will bother
you a great deal more than they bother any health
professional you consult, for the simple reason that
you live with your symptoms and with their impact
on your life every day.

You are entitled to a voice in your own health care.
No dentist or doctor is entitled to take away your
right to choose your own care and freely obtain information about it. Moreover, if a treatment or a product
appears to create symptoms of illness for you, you are
entitled to explore the situation until you find a
satisfactory answer and to discontinue using the
treatment or product if you so choose.

If you have symptoms that you believe are trig-
gered by amalgam fillings, but your dentist is scepti-
cal, one very simple route is to take one of the blood
tests for heavy metal sensitivity that are described in
Chapter 9. If you score high on mercury sensitivity
then you will have scientific evidence that amalgam
fillings are inappropriate for you. Most dentists will
not ignore a medical test showing mercury sensitivity
and will replace the fillings without argument.

If you have doubts about the accuracy of any of the quoted statements in this book, then by all means obtain copies of the scientific papers at a medical school or university library, or from an online computer link to Medline. You may also want to share the papers with your dentist or doctor.

While the specialized language of these papers is often trying for the lay reader, in most cases the conclusions can be identified without too much trouble. The bibliography of scientific papers included at the end of this book can provide a source for the information that you (and your dentist) may need.

SUMMARY

1. Mercury is a poison, and it has been recognized as such for thousands of years. The recorded literature on the subject goes back to Classical Greece. It is more poisonous than lead or arsenic—in fact, than any other metal except plutonium.

2. Technology was very primitive when mercury amalgam was introduced into this country as a dental-filling material in 1833. It was not possible at that time to demonstrate clearly amalgam's dangers, or to show scientific reasons why dentists should not use amalgam, which offered a cheap and lasting material for fillings.

3. The symptoms of mercury toxicity match the symptoms of a number of widespread present-day illnesses (fatigue = chronic fatigue syndrome; gingivitis = periodontal disease; depression; etc) as listed in both general and scientific encyclopedias and standard textbooks on toxicol-

ogy. This suggests that many of these modern illnesses, whose causes remain somewhat mysterious, may be connected to the widespread use of amalgam fillings.

4. Most dentists are not aware of the substantial body of solid scientific research that already exists on mercury toxicity from dental fillings because most of the research has been done by scientists in fields widely distant from dentistry.

5. Scientific truths require validation. It is not enough for a person or an organization to say that a statement is false, without offering documented research to verify that claim.

6. There is no documented, peer-reviewed scientific research which shows that mercury amalgam is safe. There is a great deal of documented, peer-reviewed scientific research which shows that mercury amalgam is toxic and unsafe.

7. The EPA requires that mercury left over from dental fillings be handled with extreme caution and treated as toxic waste. It is not logical to suppose that a substance which is a toxic waste once it is outside the mouth has been non-toxic while it was in the body.

8. There is no known safe level of mercury for human beings.[19] The World Health Organization issued a formal statement to this effect in 1992. The mercury present in your tissues is a toxin, regardless of whether there is a lot of it or a little. Because mercury is a toxin it interferes with your functioning to some extent, even if you have not yet experienced identifiable symptoms.

PART TWO

The Scientific
Research

CHAPTER 3

The Lorscheider-Vimy Experiments

The most crucial research in the saga of dental amalgam began in 1983, when a Canadian dentist, Murray Vimy, D.M.D., became curious about the stability of the mercury in amalgam fillings.

Vimy practices in Calgary, Alberta, where he is also a member of the University of Calgary Medical School faculty. The veteran of many discussions about dental amalgam's stability, he finally decided to settle the arguments by finding out for himself. He bought some equipment for measuring mercury vapor in the air inside the mouth and set up an initial study, testing a number of patients with amalgams under a variety of circumstances—resting, after chewing or rubbing the fillings, etc.) The resulting readings were much higher than Vimy expected—high enough to be quite troubling.

Vimy's next step intellectually was to present the results to a group of colleagues at the medical school to get their feedback. He enlisted a friend on the faculty to pull together a group of faculty members in different research areas to hear a presentation of his data in early 1984.

In the audience at this first presentation was Fritz Lorscheider, Ph.D. A Wisconsin native and a fetal physiologist, Lorscheider had been recruited when the University of Calgary Medical School was founded some 14 years previously. Lorscheider's interest was piqued by Vimy's data, which were both fascinating and disturbing. After the session, Lorscheider offered to look over the study and give Vimy some more detailed comments.

Lorscheider knew about mercury's toxic properties, of course—but neither he nor his colleagues had the remotest idea that mercury might be an ingredient in that ubiquitous silvery dental-filling material. He was thunderstruck at the notion that there might be mercury fillings in his own mouth. Later, as a result of their collaboration, Vimy, Lorscheider, and a number of other medical school faculty members had their amalgam fillings replaced. Vimy no longer uses amalgam in his practice.

Lorscheider encouraged Vimy to pursue the results of the first study on mercury vapor emissions from amalgam fillings. An earlier published study by Svare and co-workers at the University of Iowa in 1981[20], which had shown that it was possible for some mercury to escape from amalgam fillings, had essentially obtained the same results. As a result of their conversations, Vimy and Lorscheider began working together, designing a series of experiments that have rarely been equalled in their elegance and their precise results.

PROVING MERCURY'S INSTABILITY

The first task at hand was to determine whether the mercury could escape from the fillings in a quantity large enough to be significant.

In a 1985 study[21] Lorscheider and Vimy demonstrated unequivocally that mercury vapor is continuously released from amalgam fillings in measurable quantities. Measurements of air in the mouths of people with amalgam fillings showed that after 10 minutes of chewing gum, the amount of mercury vapor released from fillings was six times higher than when no chewing had taken place. During thirty minutes of continuous chewing, the mouth air mercury vapor remained high; after chewing stopped the amount of mercury in the mouth air slowly declined to pre-chewing levels over a 90-minute period.

The researchers also observed that brushing the teeth with commercial toothpaste stimulated the release of vapor from amalgam surfaces, at approximately the same higher rate as gum-chewing and for the same time periods.

PROVING MERCURY ABSORPTION IN THE BODY

Next Lorscheider and Vimy decided to try to find out whether the mercury vapor from the fillings was taken into the body, and if it was, to see what happened to it there. For this experiment, their team used dental amalgam made with the normal ingredients and proportions, but with mercury that was radioactively tagged.

Six sheep were each given twelve of these radioactively tagged fillings, on the top, biting surfaces of their molar teeth (the large back teeth on which most heavy chewing is done.) To ensure that the test was fair, the scientists "over-carved" the fillings—they

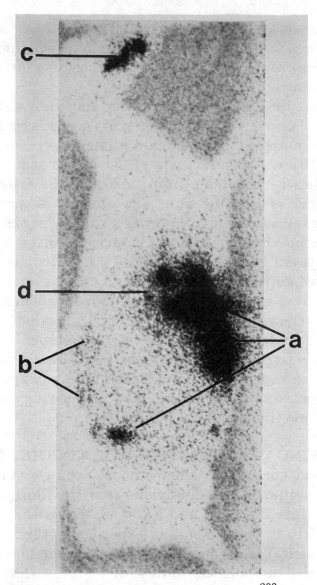

Figure 3.1 Right lateral image of amalgam ^{203}Hg distribution in the intact sheep, after removal of the dental
amalgams, with superimposed transmission scan showing
the body contour. The greatest concentrations of ^{203}Hg are
in the gastrointestinal tract *(a)*, kidneys *(b)*, and in the gum
and alveolar bone of the jaws *(c)*. Liver activity *(d)* is
obscured by large quantities of Hg in the gut on this image.

Table 3.1 Concentration of amalgam Hg in sheep tissues 29 days after placement of dental amalgam fillings.

Tissue	ng Hg/g
Whole blood	9.0
Urine	4.7
Skeletal muscle (gluteus)	10.1
Fat (mesentery)	0.9
Cortical maxillary bone	3.6
Tooth alveolar bone	318.2
Gum mucosa	323.7
Mouth papilla	19.7
Tongue	13.0
Parotid gland	7.8
Ethmoturbinal (nasal) bone	10.7
Stomach	919.0
Small intestine	28.0
Large intestine	63.1
Colon	43.1
Bile	19.3
Feces	4489.3
Heart muscle (ventricle)	13.1
Lung	30.8
Tracheal lining	121.8
Kidney	7438.0
Liver	772.1
Spleen	48.3
Frontal cortex	18.9
Occipital cortex	3.5
Thalamus	14.9
Cerebrospinal fluid	2.3
Pituitary gland	44.4
Thyroid	44.2
Adrenal	37.8
Pancreas	45.7
Ovary	26.7

scooped them out a little more than would have been done in normal dental work, so that the filling was slightly concave and the chewing pressure on these filled teeth was lighter than usual.

Three days after the fillings were inserted, the sheep began excreting mercury in their droppings. After the sheep had had their fillings for 29 days, full-body X-ray photographs were taken of the sheep.

The X-ray pictures showed that **the radioactively tagged mercury from the fillings was present everywhere in the sheeps' bodies.** It was found in the heaviest concentrations in the gastrointestinal tract, and next in the kidneys, liver, and brain. Heavy concentrations were also found in the jawbones, the gum tissues and the lining of the trachea.

Lorscheider and Vimy's article on this study was published in a prestigious scientific periodical, the **FASEB Journal**.[22] The article included the x-ray photographs of the sheep, in which the mercury scattered throughout the body is clearly visible as clusters of little black dots on the photographic plates. In the mouth and gastrointestinal tract, so many black dots had accumulated that they formed large patches of solid black.

In the analyses of the mercury content of different organs and tissues, several things stand out.

First of all, the levels of mercury in the blood and urine are not particularly high. This is useful information because blood and urine tests were once commonly thought to be valid ways of measuring how much mercury the body contains. Judging from the Lorscheider/Vimy experiments, blood and urine tests bear little relationship to how much mercury is pre-

sent in body tissue. Samples of whole blood drawn
from the sheep contained 9.0 ng per gram of mercury,
urine 4.7 ng per gram. But the kidney contained
7,438 ng/mercury per gram[23]—740 times more
than in whole blood, and 1,487 times more than in
urine. Feces contained **4,489.3 ng/mercury per
gram**—448 times more than blood, and almost 1,000
times more than urine.

Other organs which had substantial amounts of
mercury were the stomach **(929 ng/g of mercury)**,
the liver **(772.1 ng/g of mercury)**, the bone in which
the teeth were mounted **(318.2 ng/Hg/g)**, the gum
tissue **(323.7 ng/Hg-g)** and the tracheal lining **(121.8
ng/Hg-g)**.

There were smaller amounts in the glands and in
the brain itself; these organs contained amounts of
mercury two or three times larger than the blood and
urine totals.

From the distribution of the mercury, it is easy to
see what the body is trying to do. There are large
concentrations of mercury along the pathway
through which mercury is inhaled and swallowed.
There are far larger concentrations of mercury in the
excretory organs—the kidneys and the gastrointestinal tract—than in the non-excretory organs. The
body is trying to get rid of this poisonous substance
by flushing it out as quickly as possible.

Later studies showed that elimination is hindered
by the interaction of the mercury itself with body cells
and processes. For example, the mercury which finds
its way to the kidneys appears to remain there for a
long time, exiting the body only in very small quantities
by way of urinary excretion. The feces thus become the
main avenue of excretion for mercury.

The article concluded with a summary of their views:

> **Our laboratory findings in this investigation are at variance with the anecdotal opinions of the dental profession, which claims that amalgam tooth fillings are safe. Experimental evidence in support of amalgam safety is at best tenuous. From our results we conclude that dental amalgams can be a major source of chronic Hg exposure. As it has been estimated that in North America 100,000 kg of amalgam are used each year in dentistry, continuing research in this area is essential and may have an effect on public health.[24]**

After its publication, this study was criticized by the dental associations because sheep have different chewing patterns from those of human beings. Sheep tend to masticate what they eat several times, so critics contended that the longer, heavier chewing patterns of the sheep could have biased the study by showing more mercury migration than would have been true for humans. These were also points raised by the authors of the study.

Undaunted, Lorscheider and Vimy mounted another study. This one was performed with a monkey, which as a primate has a chewing pattern very close to that of humans. This second study showed similar results, and was even more interesting.

As was the case for the sheep, the mercury had migrated throughout the body of the monkey within the 28 days of the study. But in the monkey, mercury was present in the jawbone (**7,756.1 ng/Hg/g**) and gums (**4,190.4 ng/Hg/g**) in astonishing quantities—compared with deposits in the sheep jawbone averag-

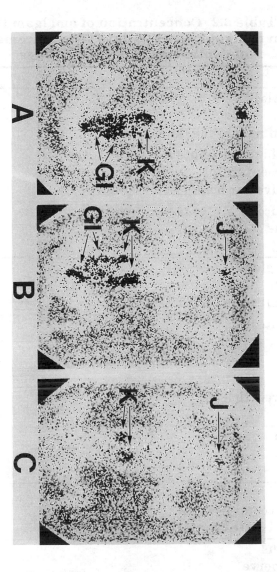

Figure 3.2 Whole-body image scan of amalgam ^{203}Hg localization in a 7-year-old male monkey (M. fascicularis) after removal of dental amalgams. A superimposed transmission scan with a ^{57}Co source outlines the body contour. *A)* Ventral image; *B)* dorsal image; *C)* dorsal image after removal of the gastrointestinal tract. J, jaw; K, kidneys; GI, gastrointestinal tract.

**Table 3.2 Concentration of amalgam Hg
in monkey tissues 28 days after placement
of dental amalgam tooth fillings.**

Tissue	ng Hg/g
Whole blood	5.8
Urine	17.7
Synovial membrane (knee joint)	31.6
Skeletal muscle (gluteus)	1.9
Fat (mesentary)	0.0
Tooth alveolar bone	7756.1
Oral mucosa	86.6
Gingivae	4190.4
Tongue	253.3
Parotid gland	1.6
Stomach	18.4
Small intestine	68.9
Large intestine	983.1
Colon	482.7
Bile	243.1
Feces	3490.2
Heart (ventricle)	6.6
Lung	15.0
Trachea	12.6
Kidney	3053.5
Liver	133.1
Spleen	15.6
Frontal cortex	7.2
Occipital cortex	12.6
Thalamus	9.9
Sciatic nerve	0.0
Spinal cord	0.0
Cerebrospinal fluid	1.9
Pituitary	83.6
Thyroid	4.1
Adrenal	31.3
Pancreas	15.6
Testes	12.7

ing **318.2 ng/Hg/g** and in sheep gum tissue, **323.7 ng/Hg/g**.

In other words, the amount of mercury in the smaller jawbone of the monkey was proportionately 20 times more than the amount in the sheep's jawbone; and the amount in monkey gum tissue was 13 times higher than in the sheep.

In the monkey kidney, mercury accumulations of **3,053.5 ng/Hg/g** were measured, and in monkey feces **3,490.2 ng/Hg/g**, about half and three-quarters the amounts for sheep kidneys **(7,438 ng/Hg/g)** and feces **(4489.3 ng/Hg/g)**.

There were also significantly larger quantities of mercury in the monkey's large intestine, colon, bile, and tongue. The suggestion was given from comparison with other studies that longer exposure results in higher accumulations of mercury. The scientific team concluded:

> **Preliminary reports on two recent investigations indicate that kidney function and intestinal and gingival flora populations are significantly altered when animals are exposed to amalgams. Hg dose accumulations were delivered from 12-16 occlusal amalgam fillings for 1-2 months after placement.**[25]

One other conclusion suggested by the comparison of the two experiments is that different species accumulate mercury at differing rates in specific body parts. Despite the fact that the critics of the first experiment apparently assumed that the quantities of mercury accumulated would be smaller in monkeys than in sheep, **in important respects the studies showed just the opposite.** The monkeys absorbed much larger quantities of amalgam in certain areas than did the sheep. They retained far more mercury in their gum tissues and tongue, jawbone, large intestine, and in their bile. They had smaller, but still enormous, quantities of mercury in the kidneys and g.i. tract.

Humans are primates and thus may be more similar to monkeys in the amounts and locations of mercury accumulation. Not enough animal tests have been done to understand fully the differences. But the results of these experiments are extremely provocative, given the high percentage of humans who have mercury amalgam fillings.

MERCURY AND THE KIDNEYS

Because of the large quantities of mercury measured in kidney tissues in both the sheep and monkey experiments, the Calgary scientists next decided to investigate the impact of amalgam fillings on kidney function.

Again, they started with sheep. They took six adult ewes and gave each one twelve radioactively tagged molar fillings, three in each quadrant of the mouth. The total mass of mercury in each animal came to 5,100 milligrams, that is, about 425mg of mercury per filling.

Two control sheep received fillings of glass ionomer, a material which does not contain any mercury.

In addition, in this experiment the fillings were left in place longer, so that a comparison was possible between one month's and two months' accumulation of mercury.

Kidney tests (renal clearance tests) were given to each animal before they received the mercury amalgam fillings, and then again thirty days and sixty days afterward. The two control sheep were tested 30 days after they received their amalgam-free fillings of glass ionomer.

At 30 days after the insertion of the amalgam fillings, **all six animals showed a decline in kidney function of 54%**. Within 60 days, kidney function had dropped **60%** from its original level. Sodium concentration in the urine tripled (from 24.8 to 82.2), and conversely albumin (protein) concentration dropped to one-third of its original level (from 93.0 to 30.1). In other words, the sheep with fillings excreted three times more salt and only one-third as much protein as normal sheep. There was no change in the two control sheep who did not receive mercury amalgam fillings. [26]

The study established that mercury accumulation in the kidneys causes increased salt excretion by blocking normal reabsorption of sodium into the body through the kidney tubules. What would this process mean to a human being, in terms of functioning?

First, it would probably result in a low sodium level in the body, with the result that the individual affected might crave salt and add it to food. Because of the low sodium level, the individual might become dehydrated more easily than someone with normal salt levels.

It is well known that hypertension is one response to decreased sodium content in the blood. Low sodium levels stimulate the kidneys to release renin, an enzyme that raises the blood pressure. So the person might also be more likely to develop hypertension.

There can be other side effects. Technically, electrolytes such as sodium and potassium must be in proper balance in order for the human metabolism to work effectively. A low sodium concentration in the body can cause muscle weakness and fatigue. Electrolyte imbalance can also cause heart irregularities because the body tissues and fluids are less able to carry nerve impulses of a normal strength.

The scientists noted that:

No [tissue changes] were observable by light microscopy after the 2-month course of this study. This would suggest that the changes in [kidney] function we have observed are not due to an actual nephrotoxicity, but rather are the results of subtle subacute effects from chronic low-dose exposure. [27]

These dramatic changes in functioning occurred over a course of just two months, without any discernible tissue changes visible under a microscope. This means that mercury can cause major disruptions in functioning quite quickly and without any visible breakdown in tissue structure.

Lorscheider and Vimy's achievement in confirming beyond any doubt the instability of the mercury in amalgam dental fillings and its absorption into the body has laid a foundation for research for many years to come. It marks a major advance in the study of human health and disease. Now that we know that everyone who has amalgam fillings has absorbed mercury from them, we can reevaluate, and gain totally new perspectives on some human illnesses that so far have baffled scientists.

For a more recent review update of related research in this area see Lorscheider et al., FASEB Journal 9:504—508, 1995.

SUMMARY

Dr. Fritz Lorscheider, Dr. Murrray Vimy

1. "Silver" mercury amalgam dental fillings constantly release mercury vapor into the mouth air. They release larger quantities of mercury during chewing, and continue to release higher quantities of mercury vapor for an hour and a half after chewing has stopped.

2. Mercury begins to be deposited in the body immediately when amalgam fillings are installed. If the mercury in the fillings is radioactively tagged, it can be detected in urine and feces within several days and can be seen in large quantities on x-ray photographs of the whole body within 29 days.

3. In animal experiments, the presence of amalgam fillings in the mouth is associated with a decline in kidney function of **54% within 30 days and 60% within 60 days after insertion of the fillings**. These changes were sub-clinical—that is, *the kidneys showed no tissue changes and the animals had no overt symptoms of illness.*

4. This suggests that mercury's presence in the body can cause major damage to functioning before visible tissue changes or external symptoms of illness can be observed.

5. The use of animal tests to predict effects in humans is a standard practice in contemporary scientific research. Therefore since standard procedures were rigorously followed, these results can be assumed to be valid.

CHAPTER 4

The Link Between Mercury and Alzheimer's Disease

O ne modern illness which has caused untold human anguish is Alzheimer's disease. Every American fears it as we grow older.

A progressively deteriorative disease of the brain and nervous system, it brings with it memory loss, personality changes, the disappearance of higher mental functions, and an increasingly limited existence culminating in death.

Among the first studies done to test for a link between Alzheimer's and mercury toxicity were a series of experiments conducted by Dr. William Markesbery, Director of the Sanders Brown Center on Aging at the University of Kentucky, and Dr. William Ehmann. Markesbery and Ehmann have systematically autopsied the brains of patients who died of Alzheimers' Disease and those of age-matched control patients who died of other causes.

Their research began to show that the AD brains contained a much higher percentage of mercury than

did the brains of patients who died of other causes—
roughly twice as much overall.

Moreover, the AD brains had lower levels of the
two major minerals that are mercury antagonists—
zinc and selenium. In two areas of the brain govern-
ing memory storage, the mercury levels were particularly high and the zinc and selenium levels were
unusually low. This suggests that zinc and selenium
may have been depleted in these areas as a result of
the high mercury accumulation. [29]

Needless to say, this was intriguing. But where
did the mercury come from? The scientists set out to
identify its source. One obvious possibility was that
it came from food, such as tuna and other contaminated fish. But there was simply too much mercury
in the brain tissue to have come from dietary sources.
Moreover, the subjects had not held jobs which would
have led them to absorb mercury in the course of their
work. How could ordinary people of this age have
been exposed to so much mercury? The mercury in
dental fillings provided an obvious solution

The same scientific team demonstrated in an
earlier experiment that in persons who died of AD, a
brain area that transmits memories and sensations
to the higher brain—the nucleus basalis of
Meynert— had mercury levels that were four times
higher than that of the controls (39.3 versus 8.9 ng/g
wet weight.) [30]

It has already been firmly established, both by
modern scientific research and by the records of history, that mercury is a potent toxin for the brain and
nervous system. The link between mercury and
Alzheimer's Disease, therefore, is quite logical. The
presence of so much mercury in the mouth, in close
proximity to the brain, and the fact that mercury

vapor is constantly released from amalgam dental fillings, provides constant exposure of the brain and nervous system to mercury.

People differ broadly in their sensitivity to all substances, including toxic ones; some are hypersensitive and have virtually no defense against a particular substance; others have well-developed and highly efficient physiological coping mechanisms. It is reasonable to suppose that in a population where the majority of adults are continually exposed to mercury in the mouth over long periods of time, some would develop brain and nervous system disorders as a result.

In addition to the Markesbery studies showing mercury in the brains of AD victim, a California dentist has shown that mercury is present in the brains of people who have amalgam fillings but who do NOT have Alzheimer's. In a study published in 1987[31], David Eggleston, D.D.S. measured the amount of mercury in the brain tissues of accident victims and correlated it with the number of surfaces of dental amalgam fillings. The results: compared with controls who had 0-1 amalgams, there was more than twice as much mercury in the grey matter of those with 5-14.5 amalgam fillings, and **three times** as much mercury in their white matter.

One subject in Eggleston's study was a pregnant woman who was carrying a 7-month-old fetus at the time of her death. The mother's teeth contained 14 amalgam surfaces. Both the mother's brain and the fetus' brain contained measurable quantities of mercury.

Another subject (who ultimately was not included in the final data analysis) was a 53-year-old, slightly obese white woman, whose car ran head-on into a cement pole at about 50 miles per hour. She had 30 amalgam surfaces in her mouth—and a level of mercury in brain tissue that was **approximately 1,000 times the mean level of the other subjects in the study**. Her kidney and liver samples also showed high levels of mercury.

Eggleston suggests that if this woman had survived, she would have shown symptoms of severe mercury poisoning. But it is also possible that the high level of mercury toxicity might have resulted in nervous-system problems that caused or contributed to the woman's accident—and therefore to her death.

HOW MUCH MERCURY
COMES FROM AMALGAMS?

The next question is: how could we determine that the mercury in brain tissue comes from amalgams?

One clue has been provided by the work of Dr. Vasken Aposhian and his wife Dr. Mary Aposhian, at the University of Arizona School of Pharmacology.

Aposhian's original interest in mercury toxicity focused on how to remove mercury from the body. Since the early 1980's he has been working with chelating agents—chemicals which bond to mercury molecules and allow them to be excreted.

The most promising chelating agent for mercury is a drug developed in Russia, DMPS (Dimercapto-propanol-l-sulfonate). DMPS is designed specifically to mobilize mercury, but it has also been approved as a remedy for childhood lead poisoning. It is given by capsule or by injection.

After hearing of the Lorscheider/Vimy research, Aposhian decided to see if he could find evidence for an accumulation of mercury in the body related to the number of amalgams in the individual's teeth. He reasoned that if the mercury body burden comes wholly or partly from amalgams, the amount of mercury in body tissue ought to be roughly proportional to the surface area of the amalgams in the mouth. With the collaboration of his dentist, Dr. Alter, he designed a project to test this hypothesis.

The result of this study has been the development of an amalgam score which reflects the amalgam surface area.

To find subjects for the experiment, the Aposhians placed an ad in the college newspaper, asking for male and female student volunteers both with and without amalgams. From those who responded, ten men and ten women were selected. The volunteers were told not to eat any seafood for a month and to fast the night before they came in to be tested. The next day they came to the lab and were given 300 mg. of DMPS by mouth. Then for nine hours all their urine samples were collected and analyzed by Aposhian's lab.

The results: the students who had no amalgams excreted one-third as much mercury as those who had amalgams. This suggests that in an individual with amalgams, two-thirds of the body burden of mercury comes from the person's dental fillings. [32]

BIOCHEMICAL APPROACHES

There are other approaches to Alzheimers' besides studying the bodies of those who have had it. A different strategy is to try to produce the disease in the laboratory, either in animals or in tissue cultures. Dr. Boyd Haley, at the University of Kentucky's Lucille Markey Cancer Center, has been working with the biochemical aspects of Alzheimers' by trying to determine what toxins produce the biochemical disturbances observed in AD brains.

Alzheimers' produces unusual nerve cell formations in the brains of its victims-" "neurofibrillary" tangles" (NFT's). Instead of growing into a normal shape, the cells sprout helter-skelter into a tangled snarl that is useless for transmitting nerve impulses. These nerve cells are built by the body partly from a substance called tubulin.

In one experiment, Haley tried adding small amounts of various other metals and of mercury to brain cell tissue cultures. He then measured the formation of brain cell microtubules from tubulin. It remained normal.

However, when Haley added small amounts of mercury to the brain cell cultures, along with a common food preservative, EDTA (Ethyline diamine tetracetic acid), the tubulin no longer behaved normally—it lost its ability to form microtubules.[33]

Brain cell cultures in petri dishes, however, are very different from the brain of a living organism. It was provocative that mercury and EDTA produced malformed tubulin; but it did not prove that the mercury/EDTA combination would produce Alzheimers'.

In the summer of 1993, Haley joined forces with Vimy and Lorscheider to form a study related to Alzheimer's Disease. Their first report was published in May, 1994 in *Neurotoxicology*.[34]

They first tried feeding inorganic mercury (mercuric chloride) to rats for 4-6 months. This markedly increased brain mercury levels, but the behavioral results were not as clear as they wished. One rat became extremely ill, staggering around and exhibiting what appeared to be the rat version of Alzheimers'. The other rats seemed relatively normal, "although they weren't nearly as frisky as they were at the beginning of the experiment," Haley said. Only the one ill rat displayed brain tubulin deformities similar to Alzheimers'.

Feeding animals mercury, however, is not the same thing as exposing them to *breathing* mercury vapor. Haley, Vimy and Lorscheider reasoned that because mercury vapor from amalgam fillings is absorbed into the sinuses and goes through the blood stream directly to the brain, they might obtain a stronger result by exposing the rats to mercury vapor.

The team calculated a dose of mercury vapor that would be the rat equivalent of a humans inhaling the vapor from fillings. They exposed six rats to these carefully-measured quantities over a period of 7 days to 24 days. The result was stunning: all six experimental animals treated with mercury vapor deteriorated markedly.

When their tissues were examined, **all six rats had brain aberrancies like those found in human Alzheimers' patients.**

The result was so astonishing that the team performed the experiment a second time. The results were the same. The rats' functioning deteriorated continuously over the duration of the experiment, and upon autopsy it was found that their tubulin was deformed exactly like that in human Alzheimers' patients.

In scientific terms, this experiment does not prove that mercury vapor from amalgam fillings causes Alzheimers' Disease in humans. In order to do that, evidence would have to be obtained through human studies—and nobody could ethically try to cause Alzheimer's in a human being.

However, even though this does not constitute scientific proof in the strictest sense, it is substantial enough to merit serious consideration by everyone who has dental fillings. In Dr. Haley's words, "The results of this experiment are terrifying. I'm getting the rest of my mercury fillings taken out right now, and I've asked my wife to have hers replaced too."

If inhaling mercury vapor can cause this kind of serious brain damage in animals, the chances are very good that it can do something similar in human beings. Even if mercury does not cause Alzheimer's disease, it could clearly exacerbate the condition in sensitive individuals.

How does this research relate to the Alzheimer's research community's current interest in Apo-E protein and the recent discovery of a genetic marker on Apo-E for early-onset Alzheimer's Disease?

Haley says there is a very clear relationship between the two. The protein involved, Apo-E protein, is a cholesterol transport protein; its function appears to be removing "bad" (LDL) cholesterol from the brain to the cerebro-spinal fluid, and then out of the body. Everyone has two copies of this gene, one from each parent, numbered either E2, E3, or E4. Combinations are also possible.

> If you have 2 copies of E2, your chances are only 30% that you'll get AD if you live to be 85.
> If you have 2 copies of E4, your chances of getting Alzheimer's before the age if 65 are 70%.
> E3 is intermediate between the two.

Every protein is made up of amino acid residues. What Haley found when he looked up the primary structure of the molecules is that the only difference between E 2,3 and 4 is a substitution of two amino acid residues in the basic sequence.

Apo-E2 (very protective) has two cysteines (which bind to mercury.)

Apo-E3 (moderately protective) has one cysteine and one arginine (cysteine binds mercury, arginine does not).

Apo-E4 (early-onset AD) has two arginines. Neither binds to mercury.

Haley's working hypothesis is that Apo-E2 could take mercury out of the body and decrease one's chances of contracting Alzheimer's until late life when a high mercury accumulation has built up. Apo-E3 will provide some protection, but not as much because it has only one cysteine. Apo-E4's two arginines provide no protection against mercury and may bestow a predisposition to Alzheimer's.

A PHYSICAL DIAGNOSTIC TEST

Boyd Haley has another Alzheimer's-related discovery to his credit. He has found a positive molecular marker which has the potential to become a physical diagnostic test for Alzheimers', the first such test that has been created. If progress continues at its current rate the test should be made available to physicians and the public 1997-98.

Haley found that the spinal fluid of deceased Alzheimer's patients contains an enzyme—glutamine synthetase—whose function is to detoxify the brain by lowering its levels of glutamate and ammo-nia (both substances are toxic to the nervous system.) Glutamate, in particular, constantly activates the neurons, so that they burn up from the stress of this continuous over-activity and die.

One version of glutamate is Mono-Sodium Gluta-mate, the MSG which causes "Chinese Restaurant Syndrome." People who are sensitive to glutamate become nauseated and dizzy when they eat MSG-sea-soned Chinese food because microscopic quantities of their brain cells are being destroyed by the glutamate in MSG.

Mercury is known to block the absorption of glu-tamate by certain brain cells. If the glutamate is not absorbed and its level rises and remains high, it will kill the neurons by over-activating them.

Glutamine synthetase is present in the spinal fluids of Alzheimer's patients.   It is NOT present in the spinal fluids of most non-demented individuals, who don't have Alzheimer's. Reasoning backwards, Haley believes that there must be an excess of gluta-mate in the brains of Alzheimer's patients—more than their normal supply of g.s. can handle. This results in an increased production of g.s. and its excretion into the cerebrospinal fluid, where the pres-ence of g.s. and glutamate can then be measured.

Because of this, the presence of glutamine syn-thetase in the spinal fluid could provide a physiologi-cal diagnosis of Alzheimer's, even in the very early stages when other tests are still inconclusive.[35]

Haley notes that it is possible that there are other dementias not yet tested that also cause increased production of g.s. For the moment, he has worked only with Alzheimer's.

As this book goes to press, news has been announced of another diagnostic test for Alzheimer's based on the contraction time of the pupil of the eye when exposed to a bright light. This procedure is non-invasive.

SUMMARY

1. Markesbery and Ehmann's research shows that there is a higher level of mercury in the brains of persons who died of Alzheimers. There is also a lower level of the two major minerals which protect against mercury—zinc and selenium.

2. The mercury levels are highest in several specific brain areas having to do with memory storage.

3. There is also a higher level of mercury in the brains of people who have amalgam fillings.

4. The Aposhians' research shows that two-thirds of the body burden of mercury comes from amalgam dental fillings, with only one-third deriving from food and other environmental sources. This suggests that if amalgam fillings were banned, individual exposure to mercury would be greatly reduced over a period of time.

5. The body burden of persons who already have amalgam fillings will not be immediately eliminated if fillings are removed, since mercury remains in the tissues for years after exposure. But the body burden can be reduced through the use of chelating agents such as DMPS and DMSA. If amalgam fillings were banned, however, expo-

sures would be eliminated for people who did not yet have mercury fillings.

6. Aposhian's research into the use of DMPS as a chelating agent is extremely valuable because of the need to force mercury out of the tissues, particularly for those who are already toxic.

7. The tubulin in the brains of Alzheimers' victims is biochemically aberrant and shows the highest overall concentrations of mercury, according to Dr. Boyd Haley. This connection is important, although its exact meaning is not yet known.

8. The presence of glutamine synthetase in the cerebrospinal fluid of persons with Alzheimers' Disease may provide us with the first physiological test for the diagnosis of Alzheimers' in living persons.

CHAPTER 5

The Immune System, Antibiotic Resistance and Other Mercury-Linked Syndromes

D r. David Eggleston is a quiet, soft-spoken man with a thoughtful manner. A faculty member at the University of Southern California School of Dentistry, Dr. Eggleston is also in private practice in Santa Monica and has a roster of star patients including Tom Cruise. Eggleston has also produced some startling and thought-provoking research on the toxicity of dental amalgam.

In 1984, Eggleston published a study that is haunting because of its importance and its lack of sequel.[36] Eggleston secured the cooperation in an experiment of three of his patients who were to have gold inlays to replace amalgam fillings or fill new decay in their teeth. Two patients agreed to have amalgams removed, reinserted, and removed again; another agreed to have a nickel-based crown inserted, which would later be replaced with a gold crown.

Eggleston first measured several important immune system components, the T-lymphocytes, in the patients' blood. The normal range for T-lymphocytes is considered 70–80% of the lymphocyte population. In one 21-year-old woman with amalgam fillings, the T-lymphocytes comprised 47% of her lymphocyte population. When Eggleston removed her amalgam fillings and replaced them with plastic temporary fillings, the T-lymphocytes rose from 47% to 73%—an increase of 55.3%!

Next Eggleston removed the plastic fillings and reinserted amalgam. The T-lymphocytes fell from 73% to 55% (a decrease of 24.7%).

Finally, Eggleston removed the second set of amalgam fillings and inserted gold inlays. After this procedure, the T-lymphocytes bounced back up to 72% (a rise of 30.9%).

Patient No. 3 was a 35-year-old white woman, with symptoms of advanced multiple sclerosis. After nine amalgam fillings were removed, her T-lymphocyte level rose from 60% to 71%. It is not known what other long-term results may have occurred, although obviously such information would be interesting.

Patient No. 2 was a healthy 20-year-old white male. When a composite filling was removed and replaced with a nickel-based crown, his T-lymphocytes dropped from 63% to 56.7%. They rebounded to 73% when the nickel crown was removed and replaced with gold.

Although the public is not aware of it, this nickel crown experiment is highly suggestive. Many dental crowns are formed on a nickel base. But nickel is a known carcinogen; industrial studies of worker exposure to nickel dust and alloys show that such exposure "will markedly increase the incidence of cancer."

[37] While no studies have been done on the effects of dental nickel, Eggleston's experiment suggests that nickel may also be hazardous to the human system.

Eggleston concludes,

> **An abnormal T-lymphocyte percent of lymphocytes or a malfunction of T-lymphocytes can increase the risk of cancer, infectious diseases, and autoimmune diseases. 3,8,10-16,19-22, 81, 83, 123[38]**

The depression of immune system functioning caused by the presence of either mercury amalgam fillings or nickel-based crowns in the body could thus increase the likelihood of cancer because the immune system would not be efficient enough to catch deviant cells before they had reached a critical mass. It could contribute to the development of autoimmune diseases such as arthritis and systemic lupus erethematosus; and increase susceptibility to infectious diseases, including sexually linked infections.

AMALGAM AND AUTOIMMUNE DISEASES

In a study published in the November 1994 FASEB Journal,[39] Dr. K. Michael Pollard and colleagues at Scripps University along with two Swedish scientists created autoimmune antibodies in mice by inserting bits of silver-mercury amalgam or of mercury-free silver alloy in the mices' bodies. Perhaps the most surprising result of the study was that BOTH amalgam and the silver alloy created autoimmune reactions in the mice. Some of these reactions were similar to those in scleroderma and in systemic lupus erythematosus. The researchers' conclusion is that prolonged exposure both to amalgam and to silver alloy causes systemic autoimmunity.

While this study was done on animals, the animal model is widely used and understood in scientific research, and the scientific community has wide experience in projecting what such animal study results might mean for human beings. In this case, both mercury and silver can cause autoimmune responses, including anti-nuclear antibodies (a hallmark of lupus and scleroderma.) The more numerous the bits of metal implanted, the stronger the autoimmune response.

ANTIBIOTIC RESISTANCE

Dr. Anne O. Summers, a molecular biologist at the University of Georgia, Athens, has spent twenty years of her career unravelling the mystery of how bacteria become resistant to toxic metals and antibiotics.

The problem of antibiotic resistance is one which has received increasing publicity during the past ten years. It affects millions of people each year, and it is recognized both by medical personnel and the public as a serious issue.

In the aftermath of surgery, when infection must be suppressed until the healing process has taken hold and the body's immune system has recovered its strength, the effectiveness of antibiotics can mean the difference between life and death. Over the past several decades, however, physicians have found that the occurrence of bacteria resistant to antibiotics is increasing in frequency and severity among the general population. Doctors must use larger and larger amounts as well as different types of antibiotics to cure bacterial infections

This rise in the quantity of antibiotics needed increases the cost of post-surgical treatment. In an age of distress about skyrocketing medical costs, the additional expeditures are a substantial reason for concern.

There is another aspect of the problem, however, which is more serious. Bacteria may develop resistance to a particular antibiotic, and to others of the same type. As a result, the antibiotic in use may fail to halt the infection, and a limited number of antibiotics will be left in the physician's arsenal. In particularly virulent infections, if physicians have run out of effective antibiotics and have no way to halt the infection, the patient dies.

Anne Summers' achievement, working in collaboration with teams at Calgary and Tufts, has been to show the mechanism by which mouth and intestinal tract bacteria develop resistance to antibiotics because of the presence of mercury. And in the U.S. today, the presence of mercury in the body is usually due to dental mercury amalgam—the most common source of mercury in human beings.

A native of Indiana and the daughter of a microbiologist, Summers gravitated naturally toward her father's career choice despite the fact that it was unusual for a woman at that time. She became interested in the question of antibiotic resistance in graduate school. She continued this interest through postgraduate work and appointments at several prestigious institutions, including Massachusetts General Hospital/Harvard Medical School. She is now Research Professor of Microbiology at the University of Georgia.

During the late 1970's, there was a very active scientific community in Boston that was concerned about the mechanisms and spread of antibiotic resistance. By the time Summers left Boston for Georgia, she had begun collaborative research with world-renowned antibiotic resistance expert Stuart Levy of the Tufts University School of Medicine.

In this collaborative work, Summers found that a high percentage among the bacteria of human feces were mercury resistant. The presence of this mercury resistance simply did not make sense. As far as she knew, these people (and thus their intestinal bacteria) had not been exposed to mercury. Amalgam was said not to be involved, since authoritative dental opinion at that time asserted that mercury was never released from fillings.

Consequently Summers' data were not published then because at the time she could find no clear explanation for the high incidence of mercury-resistant bacteria in these human subjects.

"Then one day in December 1989," Summers says, "I happened to open my copy of the FASEB Journal and read [Lorscheider and Vimy's] first article on installation of radiolabelled fillings in a sheep model system. I read it right through and immediately called Calgary and asked Fritz Lorscheider if he knew anything about mercury resistant bacteria. He said he'd never heard of such a thing; I said, 'let's talk.'"

That conversation was the start of a collaboration between Summers; her University of Georgia colleagues Joy Wireman, Lynn Billard and Sam Bennett; Stuart Levy and Bonnie Marshall at Tufts Medical School; and Drs. Lorscheider and Vimy at the University of Calgary Medical School.

The result of their work, published in April 1993

in the journal *Antimicrobial Agents and Chemotherapy*, showed that antibiotic resistance increases along with an increase in mercury resistance in mouth and intestinal tract bacteria.[40]

To test their theory that mercury resistance derived from fillings might in some way may be responsible for antibiotic resistance, the team installed mercury amalgam fillings in six adult monkeys. The monkeys were measured for mercury-resistant and antibiotic- resistant bacteria both before the fillings were installed and afterwards. In two of the three experiments, the monkeys' amalgam fillings were replaced with glass ionomer after 8 weeks. The monkeys' bacteria were then measured for an additional 8 weeks.

The results: the monkeys' bacteria—which were not exposed to antibiotics during the study and had not previously been exposed to mercury—developed significant resistance to mercury, accompanied by dramatic increases in antibiotic resistance after the amalgam fillings were inserted. The excretion of mercury in feces was astoundingly high during the the first few weeks after the fillings were placed (~100 ppm) and remained well above the EPA regulation levels for mercury in food (0.2ppb) for the full 8 weeks.

Moreover, the monkeys continued to excrete high levels of some mercury- and antibiotic-resistant bacteria during the 8 weeks following removal of the fillings and their replacement with glass ionomer.

Since the researchers knew from earlier studies that the DNA structures in bacteria that carry the genes for mercury resistance also carry the genes for antibiotic resistance, it follows that bacteria which have developed mercury resistance are likely to be antibiotic resistant as well.

And that is exactly what they found. Their conclusion: "silver" dental fillings foster the persistence of antibiotic-resistant bacteria in the mouth and gastro-intestinal tract.

This paper also revisits Summers' puzzling earlier data on resistant bacteria in humans. As mentioned above, these bacteria are often involved in post-surgical infections that, if unmanageable, can be fatal.

Dr. Summers' older data on humans is now under-standable in light of the animal studies.

The number of samples employed in this earlier study is impressive. From December 1977 through March 1979, the Georgia-Tufts team had collected 974 fecal samples from 640 people and analyzed them for antibiotic resistance. 56% of the group were women, 44% men. Some of the study participants were hospitalized patients at the New England Medical Center. Some were laboratory workers from eight Boston area research labs and a lab at the University of Georgia. And some were just ordinary people who wandered into the researchers' path at an opportune moment. The group was primarily adults—95.4% over 15, with a mean age of 42.7.

During the study, a subgroup of 356 persons, the majority of who had no recent exposure to antibiotics, nevertheless showed a high degree of mercury resistance as well as resistance to two or more antibiotics. In light of the animal studies, it is reasonable to consider that these people—many of whom likely had amalgam fillings—owed their highly resistant bacteria to the mercury coming from their dental fillings.

The three research teams issued a press release on April 1, 1993, describing the study's results. Reaction was cautious at first. Science News picked up the story, but there was no other immediate response. Then, nearly a month later, on April 27, the New York

Times published an article by science writer Gina Kolata entitled **New Suspect in Bacterial Resistance: Amalgam** (The mercury in dental fillings may spur resistance to antibiotics.) Kolata's article was balanced and interesting; it defined the issue in terms intelligible to lay readers. It also included comments from a number of other scientists.

Virtually the only lukewarm voice was that of the American Dental Association's spokesman, Dr. Terry Donovan, who said that the findings were inconclusive. "I don't think anyone should be concerned at the present time," Donovan said, adding, "any alternative to amalgam is considerably more expensive and doesn't last as long, with the exception of gold." He did not comment on the danger to life and health posed by bacteria which have been rendered antibiotic-resistant by being exposed to dental filling-mercury.

SUMMARY

1. The insertion of amalgam fillings depresses the immune system. Although Dr. David Eggelston did not test enough patients to produce a statistically meaningful sample, his preliminary study indicates that mercury has a clear negative effect on the immune system, varying widely according to the individual (a depression in functioning between 11% and 55 %).

2. Nickel-based crowns also cause a drop in immune system strength. Although the range was much narrower than that accompanying mercury amalgam, it was nevertheless large enough to be a concern.

3. The presence of mercury in the body stimulates antibiotic resistance among the bacteria in the g.i. tract. Dr. Summers has shown that the gene for mercury resistance is positioned next to the genes for antibiotic resistance in the bacterial genetic matter; triggering one can cause the other to trigger as well.

4. Dental amalgam is an identified factor in the widespread development of antibiotic resistance. While it is not the only causative factor, it is one we can identify now and could avoid.

CHAPTER 6

Medical Implications of Mercury Toxicity: Alfred Zamm, M.D., F.A.C.P.

There are still relatively few dentists who understand dental-filling mercury toxicity and know how to treat it. Physicians with experience in this area are even rarer. The physician who may have treated more mercury-toxic patients than any other to date is Alfred Zamm, M.D., F.A.C.P. Zamm has practiced for many years in Kingston, New York, a town located on the Hudson river about three hours' drive north of New York City.

Zamm first became aware of mercury toxicity as a result of his interest in environmental medicine. He has always had a passion for environmental literature, and began reading it as early as high school.

" But I didn't know where it was going to lead me," Zamm says now. "It led me to the fact that the biggest environmental poison facing our country is the river of mercury running down your throat. That's the number one environmental problem they could do something about *now*."

Born and raised in Brooklyn, Zamm received first-rate training at the University of Chicago Medical School, New York University postgraduate, and Bellevue Hospital. At the time, Bellevue had a world-wide reputation in patient care and as a training center. Medical students were drawn to it from all over the world because of the huge variety of cases encountered there—an exposure that gave fledgling doctors an incomparable grounding in the widest possible range of illnesses and treatments.

Zamm's training and board certifications normally would have led him to become a professor at a top-ranked medical school or a department chief at a fine hospital. But Zamm had other ideas. He was passionately interested in environmental studies. He wanted a certain quality of life in addition to a career; but a city practice would not provide that. "I wanted to go to a place where you can breathe the air and drink the water," he says. "In New York City you can only breathe *out*." He also wanted time to read, and a small-town practice afforded him that leisure. So Zamm opted to go into practice in Kingston, and still lives there today.

In Kingston, Zamm did not have either the load of responsibilities or the pressure to conform that would have been part of life at a large hospital or university. Gradually, Zamm began to realize that although he had had a superb education, there was something wrong with it that he could not define. Something had been left out; the picture was incomplete. He began to explore on his own, reading medical literature and feeling his way on instinct.

Zamm found other doctors with similar environmental interests in a characteristically innovative way. "One day I said to a salesman, 'Since you see so many allergists, is there anybody you know who's thinking along the same lines?' He said, 'Yes, there are a few people.'" Zamm took the names the man gave him, began getting in touch with the other physicians, and discovered the Society of Clinical Ecology—now the Academy of Environmental Medicine (of which Zamm, 62, has long since been a Fellow.) His small-town practice allowed him to take time off, so he formed the habit of taking two or three days at a time and going to other cities to work in the offices of doctors who interested him.

Eventually Zamm's colleagues began sending him patients that they couldn't do anything with. Usually he was able to come up with a treatment that helped, and as a result more patients found their way to him. Now his practice is almost entirely made up of difficult or undiagnosable patients from other doctors.

In the late 1960's, Zamm began to realize that for many of his patients there was another factor at work beyond the elements dealt with in conventional allergy medicine. "I became frustrated about something I wasn't sure about," Zamm says. "I had a sense that there was something missing, but it wasn't apparent. I came across some references to mercury—and my instincts told me that there was something there."

Zamm saw instantly that mercury imbedded in the body could be interfering with basic metabolic processes in such a way as to cause a huge variety of symptoms.

> **Mercury poisoning is impaired oxidation. It's like having an invisible cord around your neck that's strangling you, but you can't feel that the cord is there. [The strangulation is] biochemical, but the principal is the same: mercury reduces the amount of oxygen that you get. The**

body keeps adjusting and adjusting, but with every adjustment it gets sicker and sicker. And ultimately you will die from this.

I realized that when you were at this level of imparied oxidation, then everything else would follow: autoimmunity, inability to deal with infections, bizarre illnesses that don't make any sense otherwise. And suddenly everything started to fall into place.

Zamm sees the body's processes like that of an old factory that produces energy output, but cannot operate efficiently if it is given junk instead of clean fuel.

These environmental illnesses are due to a lack of energy packages required for the detoxification process. The detoxification process is a very expensive process, energy-wise....you handle the junk but you don't make any profit out of it. When things come into your body for which there's energy payoff, sure, you put up some energy but you get more back. But with junk, you end up metabolizing it—paying for it, and getting nothing out of it. Zero. ..You're already being strangled, you just barely have enough to get by yourself—and now you have to take care of these extra payments. You're going into debt. And that's exactly what was happening to these individuals.[41]

The first case Zamm treated was himself. He went to a local dentist and had all his amalgams removed. Afterwards, he says that he was so much more energetic and felt so much better that his administrative assistant had to have hers removed just to keep up with him.

Zamm does not believe that dental materials sensitivity tests are valid or necessary. Mercury is a poison, he says, and we don't have to perform tests to find that out—we know it already. Mercury's presence in the body will inevitably affect the body, even though it may not be causing any noticeable problems at the moment. It is a foregone conclusion, Zamm says, that if the mercury remains in your body it will be harmful to you in some way.

SUMMARY

1. Dr. Alfred Zamm's work shows that many conditions with mysterious causes, ranging from allergies to multiple sclerosis, can be cleared up if mercury amalgam fillings are removed.

2. Mercury toxicity deprives the body of oxygen. As a result, any body process that requires oxygen will be less efficient in the presence of mercury.

3. In Zamm's observation there is a connection between candida albicans infections and the presence of mercury amalgam fillings.

CHAPTER 7

The Huggins Diagnostic Center: Hal A. Huggins, D.D.S.

I n dentistry as in medicine, there are two separate tracks followed by members of the profession. One is research, a path which leads to limited involvement with patients and profound engagement in the detective work of tracking down the sources of disease. The other is clinical treatment: dealing every day with the infinite variations of symptoms presented by real living human beings, and trying to sort out quickly and accurately the best modes of treatment for all of them.

Hal A. Huggins, D.D.S. has combined both, emphasizing one or the other at different points. Huggins began his career as a practicing dentist like thousands of others. After eleven years in practice, he attended an international dentistry meeting in Mexico City in 1973, that forever changed his life and his career. In Mexico City Huggins made the acquaintance of a Brazilian dentist named Dr. Olympio Pinto.

Pinto's father had also been a dentist. The senior Dr. Pinto once read somewhere in an old journal that amalgam fillings could cause disease, so he decided to try removing amalgams from sick patients to see whether there was any change in their condition. To his satisfaction, patients with leukemia and various neurological diseases improved to the point of recovery.

When Olympio Pinto came to the U.S. in the 1960's to earn a post-doctoral Master's degree at Georgetown university, his choice of a thesis topic was the illnesses caused by dental amalgam. Pinto's professors were very interested in the subject until one day they received visits from scientists at the National Institute of Dental Research. Following that visit Pinto's advisers suddenly decided that Pinto had to choose a different topic.

Pinto wrote an alternative thesis and received his degree, but he went back to Brazil determined to find out himself how removing amalgams affected serious diseases. At this point he has probably removed and replaced more amalgam fillings than anyone else in the world.

During their conversation in Mexico City, Pinto spent hours passionately trying to convince Huggins that mercury was poisonous and that mercury amalgam fillings are toxic. Huggins, furious, refused to concede. He went back to Denver feeling that "My whole dental education and my first eleven years of practice were now challenged."[42]

Determined to prove Pinto wrong, Huggins began taking blood chemistries of patients before and after removal of amalgam fillings, and following the patients for some time afterward. The results were surprising, because they involved "patients diagnosed with incurable illnesses who were improving."[43] Huggins' efforts to inform the leaders of dentistry about this were successful only in drawing down upon himself harassment and persecution.

Huggins worked for some years to perfect his technique and maximize the help that could be offered to victims of different illnesses. He found responsiveness among a number of illnesses considered terminal or irremediable: leukemia, lymphoma, multiple sclerosis, lupus, arthritis. He has even obtained positive responses in treating some cases of Parkinson's, Alzheimers and ALS.

Huggins' practice grew into a state-of-the art clinic, with three assistant dentists, a resident M.D., access to chiropractic adjustments and crainio-sacral therapy, nutritional counseling and detoxification procedures available under the same roof. A blood test for dental metals sensitivities provides information on which products can safely be used for given patients. It provides a 30-page computerized report which patients can use in their home cities if they cannot travel to Colorado Springs.

Huggins has played a major role in raising awareness of amalgam's toxicity both for clinicians and for researchers. As a result, he has suffered a great deal of criticism from traditional dentistry, which was and remains profoundly uncomfortable about the contemporary crescendo of research demonstrating amalgam's toxicity.* It is to Huggins' credit that he has persisted despite the very painful experiences his candor has attracted to him.

---

* In late 1995 Huggins decided to close his clinic because of persistent harassment; but the laboratory and testing facilities remain open.

SUMMARY

1. Hal A. Huggins' work in clinical treatment indicates that a wide range of modern illnesses can be helped or even cured by removing amalgam fillings and any other toxic dental metals from the mouth, followed by detoxification treatment.

2. These results, obtained over more than two decades in treating thousands of patients, are still denied by establishment dentistry.

PART THREE

Mercury and Your Health

CHAPTER 8

How Can I Tell
If I'm Mercury Toxic?

Mercury amalgam fillings are inserted in the mouth—a major opening through which both air and food enter the body. The mercury vapor released by these fillings, and mercury molecules detached by chewing, are constantly inhaled and swallowed.

Once mercury is inside the body it becomes involved in the body's biochemical processes. A mercury atom can attach itself to any substance it encounters if the substance has a receptor site that fits. The mercury then "hitchikes" on existing compounds and interferes with their operation simultaneously. It's a little bit like having an unruly houseguest who ensconces himself in your home, messes up the kitchen, stops up the sinks, short-circuits appliances, leaves clothes and books strewn all over the house, constantly asks you to go out of your way, and wreaks havoc with the daily life of the hosts, all the while behaving as if he has more right to be there than you do.

The most obvious symptoms of mercury toxicity form a **symptom trail** along the immediate pathway

taken by the mercury vapor and particles: upward
from the mouth into the nose and sinuses, and then
to the brain and nervous system; downward to the
throat and larynx and into the lungs, from which it
is carried first to the heart, then circulated to the
other organs. The blood stream transports the mercury into body areas more remote from the digestive
tract, such as the arms, legs and skin.

Mercury mixed with saliva and food is swallowed
and absorbed by the digestive tract. From there the
blood stream transports it to other organ systems,
muscle tissue, and the skin. Part of this mercury
remains in the digestive tract tissue, and some also
remains in the kidneys.

Individuals differ greatly in their particular combination of symptoms in response to the same toxic
substance. Both genetic and lifestyle differences
among individuals may play a role in this.

We will trace the long chain of mercury-related
illnesses along this symptom trail, since doing so high-
lights the logical connection between the mercury's
source in the mouth and the symptoms produced along
the pathways of inhalation and swallowing.

1. Mouth, Teeth and Gum Tissues

The symptoms of mercury toxicity most often experienced in the mouth are **gingivitis**—an old-fashioned
name for periodontal disease, with bleeding, red,
sore, or sensitive gums—and **frequent cold sores**.
If you are highly sensitive to mercury you may have
more extreme symptoms, like abcesses. Pain in the
tissues of the mouth and tongue can likewise be a
reaction to the presence of mercury.

Gingivitis is listed in Goodman and Gilman and

in all of the encyclopedia articles on mercury cited in Chapter 2 as a symptom of mercury poisoning. This suggests in very clear terms that the contemporary epidemic of periodontal disease may be mercury-related. Research shows that the mercury from fillings is heavily deposited in the mouth tissue and jaw bone, especially in primates; those deposits could quite plausibly be destructive to gum tissue.

Mercury toxicity can actually cause the deterioration of the jaw bone, so that the teeth become loose and cannot be supported. At this point tooth implants, bridges, or false teeth may be required.

Small black spots where amalgam has been absorbed and accumulated in one spot on the gum and mouth tissues are called "amalgam tatoos." A metallic taste in the mouth can also be a product of amalgam fillings.

2. The Sinuses

Inhalation of mercury vapor often produces constantly stuffy sinuses. The usual medical explanation of stuffy sinuses is that they are due to allergies. But if the sinuses are inflamed because of mercury absorption, treatments designed for ordinary sinus conditions will be effective only temporarily at best. Once the medication wears off, the sinuses will become congested again. Recurrent infection of the sinuses is also sometimes found as a response to the mercury vapor released from amalgam fillings.

3. Brain and Nervous System

Mercury is a neurotoxin; it has a particular affinity

for the nervous system. It remains in brain and nervous system tissue longer than in any other type of tissue. Scientists commonly express the duration of certain conditions in terms of half-lives. The half-life of mercury in nerve and brain tissue is estimated to be approximately 18 to 22 years.[44] The simplified meaning of this is that any mercury absorbed into your nervous system will be there for a long time. It will require many years under ordinary circumstances to be completely excreted.

Mercury vapor from the mouth rises into the nasal cavity and the sinuses, where it is absorbed through the mucous membranes into the blood stream via the thick bed of capillaries underlying the mucuous membranes. From there mercury is carried directly to the brain.

This is not, however, the only way in which mercury is transported from the mouth to the brain. In a study performed by a Swedish scientist, Arvidson, **mercury that was injected into the tongue of a rat was carried by the nerve itself up to the brain**[45]—where it was later found in the brain region related to the tongue.

This horrifying example raises the possibility that the nerves of the mouth, tongue and jaw themselves transport the mercury they absorb to the brain. Do nerves in other bodily locations show this tendency as well? We don't know—but given the fact that such large mercury deposits are found in so many American mouths, it is terrifying enough that the nerves in the mouth can do this.

The neurological symptoms produced by mercury toxicity include dizziness and vertigo (with no other apparent cause;) loss of the sense of balance; inner ear problems; trembling of the hands and arms (medically termed "tremor"); or in severe cases, trembling of the whole body.

Some symptoms of mercury poisoning are perceived by others as personality failings rather than neurological symptoms. For example, the inability to concentrate is a very noticeable effect of mercury poisoning. So are unusual fearfulness; impulsiveness; irritability and bad temper; forgetfulness; and depression.

The feeling that your mental processes are slowing down, or that your mental or physical reactions are slower than usual, can be due to mercury toxicity. Sometimes this is accompanied by physical clumsiness—stumbling against objects which normally one would have missed, dropping things, falling—in other words, inadequate control of one's leg, foot or hand movements.

Aphasia - difficulty in speaking or in getting the right words in the right places in a sentence - is also a frequently remarked symptom.

Even extremely small amounts of mercury can have an impact on the delicate processes of the brain and nervous system—the body's all-important control center. A 1972 study by Chang and Hartman showed that if less than one part per million of mercury ions are absorbed into the bloodstream, the blood-brain barrier can be impaired within a matter of hours, permitting entry into the brain of substances which would otherwise have been barred.[46]

Another scientific team (Yoshino et al, 1966) observed that after mercury absorption, there is a greatly reduced incorporaton of amino acids into brain tissue. This was confirmed by other scientists.[47]

There are cases on record in which mercury appears to be causally related to cases of Multiple Sclerosis, Amyotropic Lateral Sclerosis (ALS), and Parkinson's Disease, whether through inhibition of neurotransmitters or through directly affecting the nerves and the brain.

5. Eyes and Eyesight

One of the most interesting accounts of the impact of mercury on vision was published in the September 1983 Journal of Orthomolecular Psychiatry (Vol. 12, No.3) by Jaro Pleva, a Swedish chemist whose doctorate is in corrosion chemistry.

Pleva began experiencing symptoms of fatigue, stress and anxiety, accompanied by irregular heartbeat and visual disturbances, after having had a gold bridge installed in his mouth while amalgam fillings were still present. Several visits to doctors showed that all his medical tests were normal except for slightly elevated cholesterol levels.

"Since no doctor could help me," he writes, " I decided to try to find the cause for myself." Because he is a corrosion chemist, he examined his mouth and saw that the surface of the one amalgam filling actually in the gold bridge had become extremely corroded in the short period since the bridge was installed. This suggested to him that the addition of the gold bridge to a mouth already bearing a number of amalgam fillings had set up conditions in which the mercury fillings began to corrode.

Pleva's visual symptoms included retinal bleeding, dim vision (especially after exercise) and slow and poor accommodation when going from light to dark and vice versa.

Other symptoms he listed were:

- Inability to fix gaze, uncontrollable eye movements.

- Eyes drawing to one side.

- Geometric figures in the visual field, migrating in a few minutes from the periphery and slowly disappearing.

- A "film" over the eyes

- Dry eyes.

- Arcus senilis; a gray ring around the cornea (Permanent.)

Sam Ziff notes that "progressive restriction of the visual fields, often progressing to blindness, has been reported repeatedly in almost all significant exposures of humans to methyl mercury." [48]

Hal Huggins, D.D.S., notes in the first edition of his book, *It's All In Your Head*[49] that Doty Murphy M.D. has found black spots and streaks occurring in the retinas of patients with amalgam fillings, similar to the amalgam tatoos sometimes found in the mouth. In Murphy's observation when amalgams are removed the black spots begin to disappear.

6. Ears and Hearing

Hearing loss is a classic symptom of mercury poisoning. The ears are connected to the mouth by the eustachian tubes. Inhaled mercury vapor can pass directly through the eustachian tubes into the middle ear, where it is absorbed into tissue and blood vessels.

A study by Amin-Zaki et al found that "impaired hearing to complete deafness was detected in more than 33% of the affected adults and 50% of the affected children during the 1971 Iraqi epidemic of methylmercury poisoning." [50]

7. Throat

Frequent sore throats or hoarseness can result from chronic mercury vapor exposure from amalgam. If an individual is extremely sensitive to mercury, the constant inhalation of mercury vapor released from fillings can irritate the larynx and the lining of the throat and bronchial tubes. Recurrent attacks of laryngitis, asthma or bronchitis can be mercury-linked, as can chronic asthma.

8. Bronchial Tubes and Lungs

Asthma can be an allergic reaction to mercury vapor inhaled into the throat and lungs. Since antibiotic resistance has been traced to the absorption of dental amalgam mercury into bacteria in the gastro-intestinal tract, it is conceivable that TB bacilli may be rendered antibiotic-resistant in some similar way, through the exposure of microorganisms in the lungs to mercury-vapor bearing air.

9. Heart

The best source of information on how mercury affects the cardiovascular system is a book that was written by Orlando, Florida dentist Michael Ziff, who led a healthy life but suffered a moderate heart attack at age

41—apparently because of his absorption of mercury from his own dental fillings and from placing amalgam fillings in patients. **THE MISSING LINK? A PERSUASIVE NEW LOOK AT HEART DISEASE AS IT RELATES TO MERCURY,** is based both on the existing scientific research on mercury and on the author's own experiences.

Dr. Michael Ziff had a thriving conventional dental practice, using mercury amalgam for most of his patients' fillings. In the year before the attack, Ziff's health had been deteriorating for unknown causes. Twice he had been hospitalized because he "became weak, grew dizzy, experienced nausea, and lost consciousness."[51] He had also had high blood pressure for a number of years.

There was no obvious cause for Dr. Ziff's condition. His diet had been "impeccable"; the Ziffs did not use caffeine, sugar or refined carbohydrates, junk foods or even canned foods. They took nutritional supplements and Dr. Ziff had begun cutting back on his one vice, smoking, with a view towards eliminating it entirely. His blood chemistry was excellent, with both cholesterol and triglycerides well within the normal range.

In spite of the proper diet and regular exercise, my health deteriorated. Perhaps the worst part of it was my emotional state. I had always been relatively even tempered and controlled. Progressively, I had become more irritable, depressed and subject to irrational fits of anger or moodiness. Naturally, this had placed a strain on my marriage as well as relationships with other people. To my horror I was noticing slight tremors in my hands at work, not a pleasant experience for a dentist. In other words, I

was rapidly going down hill and anxiously wondering where it would all end.

Dr. Ziff's next few years were not easy. He cut down his smoking even further, reduced his work schedule to three days a week and then raised it to four. Yet his condition remained marginal, with frequent feelings of weakness and dizziness. In the summer of 1981 he lost consciousness at a family wedding and was hospitalized. All his test results turned out to be normal. A ten-day family vacation to Bermuda had to be cut to five days because of Ziff's poor health. On returning he was diagnosed as hypoglycemic.

Several months after this aborted vacation, Ziff attended a seminar in which the lecturer mentioned that it was possible to develop chronic mercury toxicity from "silver" dental fillings.

Dr. Ziff returned home and began doing intensive research on the subject.

My only immediate sources of information were dental textbooks. To my amazement, the dental textbooks confirmed that the mercury is not locked into the amalgam fillings and that toxic reactions from mercury exposure from these fillings had been encountered in patients. This information had never been mentioned during dental school. I immediatley stopped placing mercury fillings into patients, and had my own mercury fillings removed and replaced with composites.

Dr. Ziff recovered completely from his heart disease symptoms and has been symptom-free ever since.

Ziff's points are the following:

1. It has already been established scientifically that when mercury vapor is inhaled, it travels rapidly to the heart, is absorbed by the heart, and builds up in the heart tissues.

2. There is no known single "cause" of heart disease; there are "risk factors" which seem to be associated with increased rates of heart disease, such as high blood cholesterol level, high fat consumption, smoking, stress, diabetes, obesity and lack of exercise.

What Ziff found in the research literature was unquestionable evidence that the absorption of low doses of mercury injures cardiovascular functioning.

Researchers at St. Louis' Washington University found "that mercury caused the smooth muscles in the walls of arteries to contract, thereby causing hypertension... Inorganic mercury caused blood vessel constriction and subsequent hypertension within minutes after exposure. ." (p79)

Researchers at Maimonides Medical Center in New York and the State University of New York found that low concentrations of inorganic mercury increased heart muscle contraction "by displacing calcium from its normal tissue sites. The displaced calcium then elicited increased heart muscle contractions," which also was conducive to the development of high blood pressure.

Researchers at the Temple University Medical

**School and the Harvard Medical School found
that "inorganic mercury caused actual pathological damage to the heart muscle tissue,
which in turn severely decreased heart function to a point that results in a dramatic drop in
blood pressure."**

Thus, smaller amounts of inorganic mercury
cause high blood pressure; larger amounts cause car-
diac tissue damage with low blood pressure. This
finding had also been made by I.M. Trakhtenberg in
the Soviet Union.

10. Breasts

The breasts are located on the upper part of the
trunk, just above the internal location of the lungs
and heart. Inhaled mercury vapor that passes into
the blood stream may be carried to the breasts almost
immediately. Mercury has been found in high concentrations in mother's milk, implying high concentrations of mercury in breast tissue.[52]
   This suggests the need for more research on two
counts. The first is the absorption of mercury by nurs-
ing infants from mothers who have amalgam fillings.
Given mercury's high toxicity, its affinity for the brain
and nervous system, and the vulnerable state of a
newborn's nervous system, we should be particularly
concerned about the possibility of neurological damage
from any exposure to mercury that an infant encounters from any source—including mercury from its
mother's fillings via breast milk. Neurological damage
in early infancy could lead to many later complications.
We might well wonder whether the contemporary epidemic of Attention Deficit Disorder could be linked to

the presence of mercury amalgam fillings in so many women of childbearing age.

There is speculation that there may be a link between mercury toxicity and breast cancer since mercury is a known mutagen —a substance which can cause genetic mutations during the process of normal cell reproduction. It is already suspected that there may be a link between pesticide residues in the body and breast cancer. What mercury's role might be urgently needs research clarification.

It should be noted that a connection between mercury amalgam fillings and breast cancer has not yet been made in scientific terms. Speculation about such a connection is made purely on the basis of the physical proximity of the lungs and the breasts, and the fact that other organ systems that are directly connected or physically close to a mercury intake point (the brain, the heart, the stomach and gastrointestinal tract) have been shown to be exposed to very large quantities of mercury. The recent publication of a study on the role of tight and rigid bras on breast cancer rates in **DRESSED TO KILL: THE LINK BETWEEN BRAS AND BREAST CANCER,** by medical anthropologist Sidney Ross Singer and Soma Grismaijer, adds another link to the chain of possibilities.

11. Esophagus and Stomach

Indigestion and weak stomach acid are associated with mercury toxicity. The gastrointestinal tract is one of the organ systems which absorbs the highest concentration of mercury, because the mouth and fillings are constantly bathed in saliva, and mercury is swallowed into the stomach with saliva as well as with food and beverages.

One mercury-sensitive woman known to the authors had repeated severe attacks of Helicobacter pylorii, the bacterium which causes stomach ulcers. She lost weight consistently until she reached 97 pounds, but was unable to regain weight or to stop the weight-loss process—until by chance she was tested for mercury hypersensitivity and had her fillings removed. After replacement of the fillings with non-toxic materials, her appetite gradually returned, her weight loss stopped, and her health slowly rebuilt itself.

12. Intestinal Tract

The intestinal tract is the main pathway for mercury excretion.

In scientific studies, the feces of mercury-toxic animals and humans contained extremely high concentrations of mercury.

Chronic constipation is a classic symptom of mercury poisoning. Paradoxically, recurring diarrhea is another; some individuals seem to be genetically prone to retaining mercury in the bowels while others are prone to eliminating it constantly. Bowel movements at times have a metallic smell. There is some evidence that conditions such as Crohn's Disease, Irritated Bowel Syndrome or ulcerative colitis may be associated with mercury hypersensitivity.

Candidiasis—the overgrowth of a fungus called candida albicans- is a frequent side-effect of mercury toxicity. Candida is normally present in the g.i. tract in small quantities. Antibiotic treatment kills off large quantities of "friendly" gastrointestinal tract flora that normally keep the fungus in control. As a result the candida fungus multiplies rapidly. When the immune system is weakened by the presence of mercury, candida seems to grow especially strong and virulent.

In its normal state, candida is confined to the gastrointestinal tract. Once it has begun to multiply, it produces filaments that can pass through the walls of the intestinal blood vessels and move into the blood stream.

There, the fungus has access to more and better nutrients. As long as candida is confined to the intestinal tract, it is relatively easy to control. Once it has passed into the blood stream it is said to be systemic and becomes very difficult to treat.

Dr. Alfred Zamm believes that there is a connection between amalgams and candida, and that particularly difficult infestations can sometimes be helped by replacing the amalgams. Dr. Warren Levin has found in many of the mercury-toxic patients he has treated that both systemic candidiasis and intestinal tract parasites are present, such as giardia, e. coli, and ameobiasis.

Fungi are parasitic organisms. They gain their nourishment by taking up residence on or inside a host, and then producing powerful proteins which literally **dissolve** the host's tissue. The principle is the same whether the host is a tree trunk that has become the home of a tree fungus, or a human being with systemic candidasis.

For that reason, it is not surprising that when candida becomes systemic, the human host can experience a wide variety of symptoms—aches and pains, allergies, g.i.tract upsets. The list is virtually endless.

In a person who has both mercury fillings and candidasis, it is almost impossible to differentiate which symptoms are caused by what. The blood sensitivity test can measure the degree of sensitivity to mercury, but it cannot tell which symptoms come from mercury toxicity and which are caused by the poisons produced by the fungus. Only when the candida infestation has been eliminated can the symptoms caused by mercury alone be identified.

13. Kidneys

The kidneys are second only to the bowel as a major pathway of mercury excretion—but less of the mercury gets eliminated in urine because the mercury atoms become trapped in the kidney itself. Mercury absorption is traditionally associated with glomerulonephritis, a disease in which the kidneys fail progressively.

Mercury poisoning episodes often involve frequent urination—the urge to urinate at very frequent intervals. This is because the anterior lobe of the pituitary gland, located at the base of the brain, controls the desire to urinate and is vulnerable to the absorption of mercury. When mercury has been absorbed the pituitary can go haywire, sending out the signal to urinate when only a small amount of urine is present in the bladder.

14. Reproduction

The impact of mercury on reproduction occurs in two ways: first, on the ability of the prospective parents to conceive and carry a fetus to full term; and second, on the physical development of the fetus itself.

Mercury toxicity is known to be linked to difficulty

in conception; to abnormalities in the egg and sperm which produce miscarriages, stillbirths and birth defects; and to delayed mental, speech and motor development in children. [53]

Incidents of widespread acute methyl mercury poisoning have occurred in Minamata, Japan[54] from industrial effluent dumped in the sea that contaminated fish that were part of the human food chain. In Iraq, farmers unwittingly ate seed grain that had been treated with mercury to reduce sprouting. These incidents have provoked a number of studies demonstrating injuries to the reproductive process in general and to children born into these communities in particular. While some of these incidents involved acute, rather than chronic poisoning, the Minamata Bay incident involved chronic poisoning over many years. The symptoms did not seem to differ greatly between acute and chronic poisoning.

It is interesting and heartbreaking to note that in these populations, generally the mothers usually got better over time from the effects of mercury poisoning, but the damage done to the childrens' nervous systems appeared to be permanent.

Mercury crosses the placental barrier easily and accumulates in the fetus at concentrations higher than those in the mother. A study by Tejning in 1968 showed that the concentration of methyl mercury in fetal blood was about 20% higher than that of the mother. [55] One of Lorscheider and Vimy's animal studies showed a mercury concentration in fetal tissue four times that of the mother. [56] This may be another instance in which the concentration of mercury in tissue is far higher than indicated by the level found in the blood.

Other studies have demonstrated that mercury

exposure injures the nervous system of the fetus, even at levels that are not considered to be toxic for adults.[57]

In the same vein, a recent German study of 108 children who died of Sudden Infant Death Syndrome (SIDS) between the ages of one day and five years and of 46 fetuses that had been aborted for medical reasons showed that all had high levels of mercury in the liver, kidney cortex and cerebral cortex. What is more, the mercury levels of the offspring correlated with the number of amalgam dental fillings of the mother. The children in this study had not been nursed at all by their mothers or were nursed only for a few weeks, so the mercury absorption did not take place through mother's milk.[58]

As far as we know at this time, no specific studies have been performed linking Attention Deficit Disorder to maternal mercury toxicity while the child is in utero. However it is a logical suggestion for future research.

15. Glandular System

All hormones and enzymes are proteins. Those with a readily accessible thiol (sulfur) group are easily appropriated by mercury.

Mercury has an affinity for the pituitary and the thyroid. Concentrations of mercury in those two glands have been found to be much higher than those in the kidney, liver, or brain (three organ systems which accumulate particularly large quantities of mercury).[59]

In one particularly important study done by Goldman and Blackburn in 1978,[60] rats were fed mercuric chloride and radioactive iodine in order to find out whether the mercury affected the thyroid gland's ability to take up iodine - an essential nutrient used to create thyroid hormones.

The rats were given oral doses of the mercury over 90 days and showed a reduction of the ability to take up the iodine, along with other signs of mercury poisoning. They also showed a decrease in secretion of thyroid hormones.

Next the rats were then given a 90-day rest, with no exposure to mercury. However, the depression of their thyroid function did not improve. The scientists concluded that the damage to the thyroid gland from mercury exposure was permanent. We don't know, of course, whether such damage would be permanent in human beings, but the fact that it seemed to be permanent in laboratory rats makes it an important question to be taken up in the future.

It is quite common for individuals with mercury amalgam fillings to have the **symptoms** of low thyroid hormone production (hypothyroidism), while their blood tests for thyroid function show a "normal" or "low normal" **level** of thyroid hormone. Mercury can bind to the thyroid hormone molecule's receptor sites; in so doing it renders the hormone useless to the body. There may be enough hormone present, but it is not available for use.

However Goldman and Blackburn's results suggest that irreversible damage could be done to the thyroid gland itself by the presence of mercury amalgam in the body. As a result, it is possible that any amalgam-filling wearer who has symptoms of hypothyroidism will have to take supplements for the remainder of his or her lifetime in order to have adequate quantities of useable thyroid hormone in circulation. The most effective replacement is "Armour Thyroid," small tablets made from dried beef thyroid, a form compatible to the human body. [61]

Common symptoms of hypothyroidism include: lack of energy, fatigue, depression, memory problems, irritability, low body temperature, dry skin, dry hair, brittle nails, and sensitivity to extremes of heat and cold.[62]

16. Blood

The hemoglobin in red blood cells transports oxygen and iron to the body. Hemoglobin contains 60 times more thiol than does plasma (the liquid in which the blood cells are suspended.) This rich sulfur concentration makes the red blood cells particularly fine targets for mercury ions looking for a place to bond.

A red blood cell on which a mercury ion has "hitched a ride" would be handicapped from carrying iron and oxygen to the cells. The owner might experience symptoms of anemia (caused by the body's lacking sufficient oxygen and iron in the system to produce energy.) Anemia, in fact, is a known symptom of mercury poisoning. [63]

According to Hal Huggins, D.D.S, it is relatively common for mercury- sensitive individuals to have what appears to be hemoglobin-rich blood with a high red blood cell count—along with symptoms of anemia. The combination does not make sense unless you realize that the mercury-tainted cells are not functional and die sooner than normal because of mercury's toxic effect. As a result the body keeps trying to replace the defective blood cells and ends up producing MORE red blood cells than would normally be needed. [64]

17. Immune System

White blood cells are part of the immune system and are often discussed in that category, rather than as part of the blood stream.

In numerous research studies, white blood cells (lymphocytes and leukocytes) showed considerable damage from exposure to mercury, even from amounts that were considered minimal and that did not alter the external appearance or functioning of the animal.[65] Lymphocytes cultured from humans who had been exposed to mercury showed high frequencies of chromosomal aberrations[66] chromosomal breakdown, alteration of the reproductive process, and cell death. [67]

In animal studies, **mercury-induced antibodies to the nuclei of white blood cells ("anti-nuclear antibodies") were found in 90% of the experimental animals.**[68] The contamination of the white blood cells with mercury ions led the body to identify its own immune-system foot soldiers as foreign invaders and to produce antibodies against them.

A new study directed by the Scripps Institutes' K. Michael Pollard confirms this finding and goes one step farther. Using a new, silver-based alloy which is being proposed as a substitute filling material for mercury amalgam, Pollard showed that silver also has the capacity to generate a strong pathological immune-system response, and that silver, like mercury, migrates to body tissues within a very short period of time.[69]

In short, both mercury and silver have a negative impact on the immune system. In addition, their effect is intensified when both metals are present.

Thymus and spleen lymphocytes from mercury-contaminated animals displayed a greatly reduced ability to travel to other locations in the body, suggesting that mercury may handicap the body's immunological defense system by slowing down the reaction time of its cellular troops.

18. Skin

Mercury is known to cause several conditions which involve lesions of the skin. In one, acrodynia or "pink" disease, the skin at the ends of the fingers becomes dry and rough and splits, revealing pink-colored skin underneath. This illness was common in children and infants in previous centuries because of the administration of calomel (a mercury-containing compound) to infants to calm them during teething.

Other authorities link mercury to skin disorders such as dermatitis, eczema and psoriaisis. Mercury can bind to a protein in the subdermal layer of the skin and interfere with its functioning, causing patches of skin to become dry, red and flakey.

19. Behavioral Mannerisms

A number of behaviors are associated with mercury toxicity that are not widely known or diagnosed as being connected with this condition.

Bruxism is a kind of behavioral tic: the person grinds his teeth while asleep at night. It is an acknowledged symptom of mercury toxicity, but is not often recognized as such either by doctors or by dentists. Some bruxism is so strong that the person's jaw feels sore the next morning.

"Hatter's syndrome", named after the "mad hatters" of the 18th and 19th centuries, can involve a number of different behaviors: lack of concentration; skipping from one thought to another when talking without employing normal connectives; inability to relate to other people; monologue talking, sometimes for extremely long periods of time; physical restlessness—the inability to sit still for more than a few minutes; and poor coordination (spilling and dropping things, stumbling, etc.)

"Brain fog," a symptom that is often encountered in illnesses such as chronic fatigue syndrome and fibromyalgia, is also a common symptom of mercury toxicity. Since inhaled mercury vapor from dental amalgam interferes so heavily with brain functioning, any individual who experiences brain fog and has amalgam fillings should consider being tested for mercury hypersensitivity.

Finally, if you have amalgam fillings, here is a list of frequently
encountered symptoms of mercury toxicity:

HEAD	Never (0)	Rarely (1)	Often (2)	Always (3)
Headaches				
Migraine Headaches				
Stuffy Sinuses				
Vision Problems				
Hearing Difficulties				
Memory Loss				
Lack of Concentration				
Insomnia				
Section subtotal				

MOUTH AND THROAT	Never (0)	Rarely (1)	Often (2)	Always (3)
Chronic Hoarseness				
Sore Throats				
Cold Sores				
Bleeding Gums				
Painful Gums				
Swollen Glands in Throat				
Thyroid Problems				
Section subtotal				

CHEST AND CARDIOVASCULAR	Never (0)	Rarely (1)	Often (2)	Always (3)
Asthma				
Bronchitis				
Chest Pains				
Irregular Heartbeat				
Tachycardia				
High Blood Pressure				
Section subtotal				

STOMACH AND G.I. TRACT	Never (0)	Rarely (1)	Often (2)	Always (3)
Bloating				
Constipation				
Crohn's Disease				
Diarrhea				
Gastrointestinal problems				
Irritable Bowel Syndrome				
Stomach Ulcers (Helicobacter Pylorii)				
Section subtotal				

KIDNEYS AND BLADDER	Never (0)	Rarely (1)	Often (2)	Always (3)
Frequent Urination				
Bladder Infection				
Section subtotal				

NEUROMUSCULAR	Never (0)	Rarely (1)	Often (2)	Always (3)
Muscle Tremor				
Numbness anywhere				
Section subtotal				

SENSITIVITIES	Never (0)	Rarely (1)	Often (2)	Always (3)
Allergies				
Skin Disorders				
Dry, Peeling Skin at Ends of Fingers (Acrodynia)				
Section subtotal				

METABOLISM	Never (0)	Rarely (1)	Often (2)	Always (3)
Lack of Energy				
Section subtotal				

APPARENT PERSONALITY TRAITS	Never (0)	Rarely (1)	Often (2)	Always (3)
Anxiety				
Bad Temper				
Depression				
Dizziness				
Fatigue				
Irritability				
Nervousness				
Section subtotal				

MAJOR SIGNS OF MERCURY TOXICITY	Never (0)	Rarely (1)	Often (2)	Always (3)
Metallic Taste in Mouth				
Metallic Smell from Urine				
Metallic Smell from Feces				
Section subtotal				

HAVE YOU EVER HAD		In the Past (3)		Currently (3)
Kidney Disease				
Kidney Failure				
Multiple Sclerosis				
ALS (Amyotropic Lateral Sclerosis)				
SLE (Systemic Lupus Erythematosus)				
FM (Fibromyalgia)				
CFIDS (Chronic Fatigue Syndrome)				
Section subtotal				

SCORE:

1–20 You may have some degree of toxicity, but it isn't enough for major concern.

20–40 You are somewhat toxic and should reduce your exposure to mercury and other heavy metals such as lead and cadmium.

40+ You are highly toxic. See a clinical ecologist or your regular doctor immediately.

CHAPTER 9

Having Your Fillings Replaced

There is a series of special steps that should be followed in order to have your fillings removed safely and to help your body excrete the mercury accumulated in your tissues. The most important part of this process is to replace your existing "silver" amalgam fillings with non-toxic materials. This will eliminate continuing absorption of mercury from the fillings.

However, the process of removing the fillings itself poses problems, because of the risk of inhaling mercury vapor during the drilling.

The reason for this is simple: the tip of a high-speed dental drill moves so fast that it becomes hot enough to vaporize all the mercury in an amalgam filling while the filling is being removed. The tip of the drill reaches temperatures as high as 800 F; the mercury in the fillings will be completely vaporized at 673.8 F.

As a result **both your nose and mouth must be protected by masks during the drilling, or you will inhale virtually all of the mercury in the filling while you are in the dentist's chair—and you may get worse instead of better.**

If the dental procedure itself causes you to inhale all the mercury in the filling at one time, then you have accomplished **the opposite** of what you were trying to do—and worse: you have absorbed all the mercury in the filling in a few minutes, instead of little by little over a period of years.

If you have a group of fillings taken out at one sitting without protection against inhalation, you may permanently damage your health in some respect. Large-scale unprotected removal can generate new illness or make an already-present chronic condition worse.

One anecdotal example that gives pause was an HIV-positive man whose condition was stable and who decided to have all his amalgam fillings removed in order, he thought, to protect his immune system. He had all the fillings replaced in several sittings within two weeks' time. Neither he nor his dentist realized that he should have been protected from inhalation during the procedures. Shortly after he replaced the fillings, the man's health began to decline, and he died about six months later.

From a scientific point of view, it cannot be proven that mercury inhalation during the dental procedure caused this man's decline and death; the standards of scientific proof require evidence in a very different form than is provided by one anecdotal incident. However, because of the impact of mercury in lowering the efficiency of the immune system, it is plausible that mercury inhalation could have been part of a major turning point downward.

Even polishing a mercury amalgam filling during regular dental-office cleaning of your teeth presents an inhalation danger. Polishing a filling's surface removes the "patina"—a layer of corrosion which forms on all oxidizable metal surfaces over time with exposure to air. This layer of corrosion reduces the amount of mercury vapor released from the filling, because most of the surface mercury has oxidized, leaving a layer composed mostly of other metals.

When the corrosion is removed, the newly-polished, shiny amalgam surface will emit far greater quantities of mercury vapor into your body. If you notice that you feel less well immediately after having your teeth cleaned, or if you get nauseated, tired, depressed, and out of sorts after a regular cleaning, the reason may be the greater release of mercury after polishing away the patina.

Mercury inhalation is extremely dangerous. There is no way of predicting how exposure to mercury will affect any given individual, how long it will take for the effects of the exposure to manifest, or what form the effects of exposure will take.

Inhalation can even have different effects on the same person at different times, presumably varying with the amount of mercury already absorbed, the person's current state of health, environmental conditions, and so on.

Chronic low-dose absorption of any toxin works on the same principle as filling a bucket with water using a teacup. For a long time, nothing much seems to be happening. The amount of water in the bucket rises very slowly. Gradually, however, the level creeps up, and as the teacupfuls of water continue to be added, the water level gets closer to the top. Finally there comes a point when the bucket is full— and the next teacup of water causes the bucket to overflow. As more and more teacupfuls of water are added, the overflow will continue.

No one knows how much their system can absorb

of any toxin before the overflow point is reached and they become saturated.

Some people have a great deal of resistance to a particular toxin—a very large bucket; others have virtually none—a bucket the size of a coffee mug. A blood sensitivity test is the only way of getting a rough idea what your own limitations might be. However, it will tell you only how sensitive you are at this time; it cannot tell you how sensitive you were before you were exposed to mercury or how much mercury your system has already absorbed.

If you value your health, the only sensible choice is simply never to expose yourself to mercury inhalation under any circumstances. This means removing any amalgam fillings already installed under the safest possible conditions, and never allowing any others to be placed in your mouth.

In seeking to find how sensitive you are to mercury, and how best to replace your fillings, there are several important steps you can follow.

1. Take a blood test for Dental Materials Sensitivity to determine which metals you react to and what products can be used to replace your mercury amalgam.

    This test is especially important:

    A. If you have a large number of mercury amalgam fillings and may have absorbed large quantities of mercury as a result.

    B. If you have a chronic health problem of some kind and any number of mercury amalgam fillings—regardless of how few.

    In cases of extreme sensitivity, people have been known to have severe illnesses even though they had only a few fillings. When the fillings were removed, the chronic illness disappeared. NOTE: Not everyone has this immediate response to the removal of fillings; it is more common for symptoms to diminish over a period of time, for example several months to one year.

If you decide to have your mercury amalgam fillings replaced, another type of filling material must be inserted. There are dozens of alternative materials on the market; some contain small quantites of metals. The test will identify the materials that are safe for you personally.

There are two sources for the Dental Materials Sensitivity Test.

1. The Huggins Diagnostic Center, a dental research institute founded by Hal A. Huggins, D.D.S., in Colorado Springs, Colorado, has a test kit which can be obtained for $5.00 by calling 1-800-331-2303.

The test kit contains a consent form and vials for blood samples and instructions for the lab. Your doctor will sign the form and instruct you where to go to have the blood samples drawn. The lab will send the blood samples and form by overnight mail to the Huggins Institute in Colorado Springs for processing, and a computerizd analysis will be sent to you or to your physician or dentist.

The cost of the Huggins report is $225.00. For an additional $15 you can have one copy of the report sent directly to you and a second copy sent to your doctor or dentist. The report will arrive about two weeks after the blood samples are sent off.

2. Walter J. (Jeff) Clifford, M.S. was the origi-

nal architect of the Huggins blood test. Clifford
has operated his own lab now for some years and
has continued developing and refining his testing
procedures. At the present time he uses a precipi-
tation-agglutination test, which is said to give
more accurate results than the original form of
the test.

The Clifford Test has a complete fee of $225,
including the cost of the kit and laboratory processing. It can be ordered from (719) 550-0008, fax
0009; or P.O. Box 17597, Colorado Springs,
80935. It must be ordered using a physician's
name because it is a prescription item.

The Huggins test vs. the Clifford test: There
is a certain amount of controversy about which
test is more reliable. Holistic/mercury-free dentists sometimes prefer one test over the other.
Dr. Alfred Zamm believes that the Clifford test
is superior. The Clifford test is more complicated
to obtain, however, which makes it harder on the
client who does not have an amalgam-conscious
dentist or physician. Although we do not know of
any scientific comparisons, those persons in our
acquaintance who have used the Huggins test
have been satisfied with its results. Beyond the
superficial characteristics listed in this para-
graph we do not have adequate information to
differentiate between them.

2. Find a dentist who will use appropriate safety
    precautions.
    Ask your dentist to use a rubber dam over
    your mouth and a nose mask over your nose. If
    he does not have a nose mask for patients, ask

him if you can borrow one of his fiber nose-and-mouth masks, cut it down to fit just your nose, and tape the edges securely to your face. Even better is the use of an oxygen mask, if your dentist has one available.

If your dentist is reluctant to comply, insist. If he continues to refuse, cancel the appointment—even if you have to get up from the dentists' chair after the appointment has begun—and find another dentist. Your long-term health is too important to risk by inhaling more mercury particularly if you have had a large number of fillings for many years. It is impossible to predict where your saturation point is, but if you have not yet become seriously ill, you don't want to run any risk of crossing that threshold.

This principle holds true for everyone. Being protected against inhaling the mercury vapor produced by drilling is, however, especially important for:

Children—because their body mass is smaller, so that even small amounts of mercury can affect them very strongly; and because the impact of mercury on their growth and development could affect all the rest of their lives.

Pregnant women—because mercury passes easily through the placental barrier and accumulates in the fetus. In Lorscheider and Vimy's experiments, the fetus absorbed mercury through the mother's blood stream in concentrations four times higher than that of the mother.

People who are HIV positive or who have been exposed to HIV—because their immune system is already compromised, and inhaling mercury vapor can damage it further.

People with any kind of auto-immune disorder, like arthritis, lupus, or multiple sclerosis—because mercury itself has the capacity to induce auto-immune diseases in certain cases, and will almost certainly make an existing auto-immune disease worse.

And people over sixty—because dental mercury amalgam has been implicated as one possible cause of Alzheimer's Disease.

3. Make sure your dentist knows how to work with alternative filling materials such as composites.

    Composite filling materials require more time to use and also more knowledge on the part of the dentist. If a dentist doesn't know how to manage the process correctly, there are a variety of mishaps that can occur, some of them with serious and painful consequences.

    One woman known to the authors had two fillings inserted by a dentist who was inexperienced at using composites and who did not know what kind of base or sealant should be used under the filling. The fillings proved to be extremely sensitive to heat and cold, the nerves of the two teeth began to die as a result, and the woman eventually had to have root canals in both teeth.

    The only way to find out if your dentist is experienced in using these materials is to ask him, and to ask some of his other patients as well. If your regular dentist really isn't familiar with these materials, you are better off finding a dentist who is familiar with them.

Gold is an extremely good filling material; it is non-reactive and extremely durable. The gold should be of as high a carat as possible—in other words it should contain as small an amount of other metals as possible. Gold, however, is much more expensive than composites. It is also more time-consuming because gold fillings require a two-part process: the filling must be cast from a mold the dentist makes of the hole in your tooth.

Thus there is a waiting period between drilling and the insertion of the filling of about a week's time. Despite the greater expense and the more cumbersome process, however, it is the best and most durable filling material available.

CHAPTER 10

Detoxification

I f you decide to have your mercury fillings replaced, you should also begin looking for a clinical ecologist or a holistic physician who can help you remove the mercury from your tissues during the replacement process and afterward.

As we said earlier, mercury stores in the body tissues, and it does not leave those tissues easily or willingly. As a general rule, the more mercury you have in your system, the longer it will take to get rid of it.

There are sevaral parts to the post-amalgam recovery process. The first is *elimination*. Although it's a subject most people in our society find difficult to discuss, elimination is very important for the former amalgam-wearer because of the high percentages of mercury found in the bowel in animal experiments, and additionally because of the damage mercury does to the kidneys.

The second part is the actual *detoxification*: pulling mercury out of the tissues by means of vitamins, minerals, amino acids, and chelating agents. This reduces the total amount of mercury stored in the body.

The third part is *avoiding further absorption of mercury*—from any source. This isn't as easy as it sounds; some cosmetic and household preparations contain small amounts of mercury either as a preservative or a bacteriocide.

You will need professional medical help in choosing a detoxification method and in monitoring your progress while detoxification is taking place. Expect to be involved in detoxification for a minimum of one year. The longer the mercury has been in your system, the more time detoxification may take.

A. Elimination
Most natural mercury elimination occurs through the bowel, so for mercury-toxic individuals it is extremely important to maintain good bowel movements. This isn't necessarily easy. Constipation is a frequent side effect of mercury toxicity. The presence of mercury in the body can slow down normal bowel processes almost to a halt. Some mercury-sensitive individuals have bowel diseases such as Crohn's Disease or Irritable Bowel Syndrome, which turn both digestion and elimination into painful and difficult ordeals.

If you have constipation, you will need to find preparations which do not irritate your gastrointestinal tract but which keep elimination regular. It is very important to have daily bowel movements; constipation will make you increasingly toxic until you become sick.

There are fiber preparation which can be taken daily such as Yerba Prima's Daily Fiber Formula, which maintain elimination and which also help absorb toxins in the bowel. There are also herbal laxatives such as Innerclean or Swiss Kriss, which can be taken at whatever interval is necessary for daily bowel movements. Another option is to use a bowel cleansing system for a limited period of time. There are a number of these sold through local health food stores which claim to soften and eliminate accumulated wastes. Periods of constipation may be followed by several days when bowel movements smell strongly metallic. This may mean that more mercury than usual is being released from the gastrointestinal tract into feces.

B. Detoxification
At our present level of knowledge, there is no way to measure exactly how much mercury anyone's body, or any particular organ system, has absorbed and stored, if the person is still alive. (Obviously all these things can be determined fairly easily if the person has already died!) Organ systems appear to retain mercury for different lengths of time and in differing quantities. In addition, there may be biological differences between individuals: some people may give up their stored mercury more easily than others.

However, it is possible to estimate the quantity of stored mercury by means of a "DMPS Challenge," a test which must be done by a physician. It consists of a 24-hour urine collection; then an injection or oral dose of DMPS, followed by another 24-hour urine collection. The difference in the mercury level between Specimen 1 and Specimen 2 will give your doctor a rough idea or how much mercury has accumulated in the tissues.

There are several substances which help eliminate mercury from the body. Not all are equally effective for every individual, and not much is known at this point about which are more effective or why.

1. Glutathione

2. Vitamin B6

3. Zinc

4. Vitamin C

5. Vitamin B1

6. Selenium

7. DMPS

8. DMSA

9. Activated Charcoal

Numbers 1 through 6 in the list above are drawn from *Dental Mercury Detox, 1995 Revised Edition, $3.95,* by Sam Ziff, Michael F. Ziff,D.D.S. and Matts Hanson, Ph.D. It can be ordered from Bio-Probe (see address in appendices) and is an inexpensive but priceless investment. the Ziff booklet. It is recommended that these nutrients be added one at a time, at 3–4 day intervals. This may seem like a slow pace, but it isn't. Taking too many detoxifying substances too fast can cause internal redistribution of your body's mercury stores and can actually make you temporarily sicker. The objective is to detoxify yourself and stay functional at the same time.

1. **Glutathione** is an amino acid which is centrally involved in detoxifying mercury and removing it from the body. It is recommended as the first supplement to take because any detoxification causes a shifting and redistribution of the body burden of mercury. Glutathione protects against mercury tox-

icity and can remove mercury from the brain. Dr. Ziff recommends 50 mg. three times a day, between meals so the glutathione does not have to compete with other amino acids from food.

2. **Vitamin B6** (pyridoxine) is critically involved in metabolism of the sulfur amino acids. It is also important in changing a precursor amino acid into glutathione. Dr. Ziff recommends taking one 50-mg capsule with breakfast every day.

3. **Zinc** is in the same column of the periodic table of elements as mercury, and it competes biologically with mercury. It is known as one of the two major mineral antagonists to mercury, along with Selenium. It also stimulates the production of a substance which helps remove heavy metals from the body, metallothionen.

Dr. Alfred Zamm recommends one 15 mg tablet of zinc twice a day. He observes that some of his patients report some improvement of their general sense of well-being when taking zinc. Dr. Ziff recommends one 15-30 mg. tablet daily.

Caution: In a recent experiment, demented patients who were given zinc rapidly became worse. The zinc apparently caused more rapid clumping of the amyloid plaques in the brain. As a result, if you have memory difficulties or if your dental metals sensitivity test reveals a sensitivity to zinc, it is better not to take zinc supplements.

4. **Vitamin C** is a very valuable part of any mercury detoxification program. It supports tissue repair and has the ability to bind to mercury to carry it out of the system.

The prolongued chemical stress of internal exposure to mercury can cause adrenal exhaustion and lower the Vitamin C content of the adrenal glands.

Supplementation with C will not only help to detoxify the tissues but rebuild the adrenal glands as well.

Ziff recommends 500mg with meals, 3 times per day, to begin.

Vitamin C can be taken both by mouth and intravenously. One book on detoxification, published by Queen and Company, recommends strongly that Vitamin C be taken intravenously. Many holistic dentists give Vitamin C intravenously while removing amalgams in the belief that it will help trap any mercury that is released into the blood stream during the filling removal fillings.

5. **Vitamin B1** (Thiamine) contains a sulfur group; by injection it has been used to treat mercury poisoning. Ziff notes that the symptoms of B1 deficiency and those of mercury poisoning are almost identical. He recommends a 50 mg tablet three times daily.

6. **Selenium** is the last nutrient that the Ziffs suggest be added. It has the capacity to bind with mercury to render it biologically inactive and stimulate its excretion. Tuna, for example, are not poisoned by the mercury in their bodies, because the tuna has two atoms of selenium for every atom of mercury and is therefore protected. Selenium is also protective against arsenic and cadmium. Inorganic selenium is preferable because it will not stay in the body and will be excreted.

The Ziffs recommend one 50-microgram tablet three times a day; Dr. Alfred Zamm recommends one 50 microgram tablet of selenium twice a day (or one-half dropperful of liquid selenium as it is sold by Nutricology.) Zamm says patients usually show some benefit within three days, but not always; in some cases it has taken up to three months for improvements to show.

Selenium should not be taken with Vitamin C.

7. **DMPS,** a chelating agent which was developed in Russia and is currently manufactured in West Germany, was created specifically for use with mercury poisoning. It can be taken by mouth or by injection. Injections of DMPS are are extremely effective in clearing up mercury-associated symptoms, such as dizziness, memory problems, nausea, lack of coordination, etc.

There is a cyclical response to DMPS which has been remarked by several persons who have taken DMPS to detoxify. Immediately after the dose the person feels enormously improved, a feeling which continues for approximately 3-4 days. By the fifth day the person's symptoms are beginning to recur mildly; they become more intense on the sixth and seventh days. This suggests that when mercury has been chelated out of the blood stream, after a period of several days, more mercury begins to be drawn from the tissue into the blood stream in order to maintain a kind of osmotic balance.

8. **DMSA** is a chelating agent similar to DMPS but it must be taken by mouth. It comes in tablets and has a strong sulfurous smell. We have no current information on its effectiveness. It is expensive and is said to be somewhat less effective than DMPS. Anecdotal information suggests that it may be more difficult for some people to tolerate than DMPS.

Of these two substances, unfortunately only DMSA has gained FDA approval for sale in the U.S.

9. **Activated Charcoal** is an old, familiar detoxificant, which is said to be effective in removing mercury. Because it is ingested into the gastrointestinal tract, where the largest mercury accumulations are

found, it may be a useful aid in eliminating the maximum possible mercury from the digestive tract.

C. Avoiding Further Mercury Absorption

In addition to replacing any amalgam fillings, mercury-toxic individuals should try to avoid further exposure to mercury from any source.

You will be as startled as the authors of this book to learn that many household and cosmetic preparations contain mercury, in spite of its poisonous qualities. Perhaps the assumption is that a little bit of poison won't hurt much.

Mercury's use in medical products goes back to earlier centuries when there were few antiseptics and bacteriocides and it seemed better to use mercury than to have the patient die of an infection. In the 19th century mercury was also used to drive syphilis into remission----"Two minutes with Venus and twenty years with Mercury," as a popular saying of the time went.

At this point, knowing what we do about the damage mercury does to the body, brain and nervous system, there is no legitimate reason that mercury should be included in any preparation for use on or inside the human body. Just as we would not manufacture cosmetic or medical preparations containing lead or arsenic, so we should not make any preparations for human use which contain mercury. Fortunately, because of the Federal regulations requiring manufacturers to list ingredients on packages, it is possible now to identify products which contain mercury and those which do not.

CHAPTER 11

Implications for the Future

Over the past twenty years, Americans have become highly conscious of the dangers of lead to human health. Before this awareness developed, both adults and children were often exposed to lead—but since it was not widely understood that this exposure could be damaging, it went unnoticed and largely unexamined.

When lead exposure began to be an issue, the permissible level of exposure was at first fairly high. Gradually it was amended downward again and again, as new studies showed that far smaller amounts of lead were harmful than were originally thought.

The June 1992 issue of *The Townsend Letter for Doctors* proposes that we will undergo a similar revolution in consciousness in our awareness of mercury toxicity. For 160 years enormous numbers of Americans have been exposed to mercury through dental amalgam—and in addition through medicinal and industrial uses of mercury.

We are already aware that industrial exposure is harmful and have established guidelines to prevent exposure beyond certain minimal limits. Similarly, the use of mercury-containing diuretics and antiseptics has dwindled almost to zero because of our awareness of the danger to human health of any form of mercury exposure.

In dentistry today, the same material is treated as if it is potentially extremely harmful to the dentist and dental assistants; dangerous toxic waste and an environmental hazard when discarded; and completely harmless in the mouth of the patient who is exposed to it 24 hours a day.

Behind this contradiction is an irrational combination of assumptions that are impossible to reconcile with each other. A tooth that together with its filling has been in your mouth for many years, and which becomes "toxic waste" the minute it is outside your mouth, is a tooth which has been "toxic waste" from the moment the filling was inserted. Being placed in the mouth or in a tooth does not render mercury amalgam harmless—and removing it from the mouth does not transform it into something that is toxic.

It will be many years after we stop using amalgam before we know the full range of effects on our health. It is impossible to guess at this time what percentage of heart attacks and cardiovascular disease are mercury-related; how many cases of Alzheimers' are directly linked to mercury vapor inhalation from amalgam; how much end-stage renal disease is due to mercury accumulation that gradually destroys kidney tissue until the kidney can no longer perform its functions.

Is the widespread use of mercury in women of childbearing age a factor in the epidemic of hyperactivity nnd Attention Deficit Distorder in American children? Is mercury amalgam partly responsible for the declining fertility of American men and women in their 30's?

Is the use of mercury amalgam for the dental care of welfare recipients, including children, connected with difficulty in learning, attention disorders, and antisocial behavior in those children? Is the presence of mercury amalgam linked to higher rates of cancer? Does it trigger other diseases that haven't occurred to us yet? We know that when lead and mercury are both present in the body, their toxicity is magnified many times over. Is the high lead level often found in city residents' blood combining with mercury from amalgams to produce symptoms of physical and behavioral illness? We don't know.

There is an immense quantity of research which needs to be done, all the more so because of the near-universality of exposure to mercury amalgam in the United States today. Many children who have never had mercury fillings themselves may have absorbed enough mercury from their mothers in utero to affect their development for the rest of their lives. Much medical research that has already been done may have been skewed because of different physiological reactions from those with no amalgams, a few amalgams, and many amalgams.

Twenty years into the future, we may well look back and wonder how any rational human being could ever have imagined that we could insert large quantities of mercury into our teeth and leave our health untouched. But until then, we have our work cut out for us—and, to paraphrase Robert Frost, miles to go before we will have all the answers we need.

APPENDIX A

Dentists Knowledgeable About Safe Removal of Mercury Amalgam "Silver" Fillings

CALIFORNIA

David C. Kennedy, D.D.S.   (619) 231-1624
2425 3rd Avenue   FAX (619) 231-6119
San Diego, C.A. 92101

Dr. Kennedy is an excellent clinician with many years of experience. He is also nationally know for his research and advocacy on the harmful effects of fluoride.

George Schuchardt, D.D.S.   (310) 777-2444
462 N. Linden Drive   FAX (310) 777-4694
Suite 437
Beverly Hills, CA 90210

Dr. Schuchardt is one of the most outstanding innovators in non-tox dentistry and in new methods for healing dental problems

COLORADO

Peak Energy Performance   (800) 331-2303

(Formerly Huggins Research Institute)
5080 List Drive
Colorado Springs, Col. 80919

Huggins was an American pioneer in removing amalgams and attempting to detoxify patients from mercury absorption. Like any pioneer he absorbed a great deal of criticism. He has done a great deal to publicize the problem of dental filling mercury toxicity in the U.S. and to develop new methods for the treatment of amalgam-toxic patients.

CONNECTICUT

Mark Breiner, D.D.S.   (203) 799-6353
325 Boston Post Road   FAX (203) 799-3560
Orange, Connecticut
(Train stop: Milford)

Dr. Breiner is particularly well known for his diagnostic ability, in addition to being an accomplished dentist. He has the equipment to take panoramic mouth x-rays (a full view of all teeth and gums on one film.)

FLORIDA

Frank Ward, D.D.S.   (407) 855-7380
300 Gatlin Ave.
Orlando, Fla. 32
(407) 855-6557

Milton L. McIlwain, D.D.S.   (407) 293-3185
5400 Hernandez Drive
Orlando, Fla. 32808

GEORGIA

Wayne King, D.D.S.   (404) 426-0288

1200 Roswell Road, Suite 4
Marietta, Ga. 30062

Secretary of the International Association of Oral Medicine and Toxicology.

KENTUCKY

John Hankla, D.D.S.   (606) 236-2243
Greenleaf Shopping Center   FAX (606) 238-4186
Danville, K.Y. 40422

NEW JERSEY

Dr. Paul Gilbert, D.D.S.   (732) 254-7945
123 Dunham's Corner Road   FAX (732) 254-0287
East Brunswick, N.J. 08616

Alan Steiner, D.D.S.   (201) 627-3617
35 West Main Street,   FAX (201) 627-5069
Suite 208
Denville, N.J. 07834

NEW YORK

Howard Hindin, D.D.S.   (914) 357-1595
2 Executive Boulevard   FAX (914) 357-2428
Suffern, N.Y. 10901

Edward F. Hutton, D.D.S.   (212) 645-0000
851 Fifth Avenue   FAX (212) 472-2727
New York, N.Y. 10021

CANADA

Murray Vimy, D.D.S.   (403) 266-2251
615401 Ninth Avenue S.W.   (403) 237-5759

Calgary, Alberta, Canada T2P 3C5

Dr. Vimy is one of the great pioneers in this field both as a dentist and as a scientist.

Latin America

BRAZIL

Dr. Olympio Pinto   011-55-21 537-71-74 or 3841
Rue Visconde de Ouro Preto #63   FAX 286-4763
Rio de Janeiro
Brazil 22250-180

Dr. Pinto was one of the first dentists to begin routinely removing amalgam fillings because of their toxicity many decades ago. His meeting with Dr. Hal Huggins in the 1970's had historic results through Huggins' interest and then active involvement in the subject.

ORGANIZATIONS / PUBLICATIONS:

1. The International Association of Oral Medicine and Toxicology, the scientific organization in this field, was begun in 1984 by Dr. Murray Vimy and Dr. Michael Ziff. Thirteen persons attended its first meeting in Calgary, Ontario. Today the IAOMT has 300 members in North America and chapters in several foreign countries, and holds twice-yearly scientific meetings in the U.S.

    The Executive Director of the IAOMT is Dr. Michael Ziff. The IAOMT mailing address is:

IAOMT
P.O. Box 608531
Orlando, FL 32860-8531

Requests for an IAOMT dentist in your area may be sent to the IAOMT at the address given. Please include a SASE #10 envelope with 78 cents postage with your request

The authors wish to stress that, if there is no dentist experienced in safe amalgam removal in your local area, it may be advantageous to look into the possibility of travelling to a city in which there is such a dentist. The names of experts in this area can be obtained through the IAOMT (or through DAMS — send a stamped, self-addressed envelope in either case). The difference in quality of care may more than compensate for the expenditure of time and money in making the inquiry.

2. BIO-PROBE is an organization dedicated to disseminating information about mercury amalgam toxicity. Founded by the father-and-son team of Sam Ziff, and Dr. Michael Ziff it publishes an excellent newsletter of the same name, plus an impressive roster of high-quality books.

    Dr. Michael Ziff is one of the small number of dentists who became interested very early in the mercury toxicity issue. He was himself mercury-toxic and describes the process he went through to diagnose his condition in his book on heart disease, **The Missing Line? A persuasive New Look at Heart Disease as It Relates to Mercury.**

    > BIO-PROBE
    > (407) 290-9670; FAX (407) 299-4149
    > Dr. Michael Ziff
    > Mr. Sam Ziff
    > P.O. Box 608010
    > 5508 Edgewater Drive
    > Orlando, Fla. 32860-8010

3. DAMS (Dental Amalgam Mercury Syndrome) is an organization founded by Louise Herbeck, an Alberquerque, N.M. woman, for victims of mercury toxicity from dental amalgam. In addition to publishing a newsletter, the organization is also undertaking research projects related to mercury toxicity.

   The International DAMS Newsletter costs $20. There is a basic information package that costs $10.00 for people who are inquiring for the first time. DAMS helps people locate mercury-free dentists. It sells books and occasionally provides speakers for meetings. It now has 75 chapters around the nation, 6/8 in Canada, plus sister organizations in Sweden, Finland, France, Australia, New Zealand.

   DAMS (Dental Amalgam Mercury Syndrome)
   Teresa Kaiser, Executive Director
   P.O. Box 64397
   Virginia Beach, VA 23467
   (800) 311-6265

4. Canadians for Mercury Relief (CMFR), founded by Wayne Obie, is dedicated to abolishing the use of mercury in dentistry. Their first action, in 1997, was to file a lawsuit against the Canadian FDA, Health Canada. New members are welcome; join by sending a contribution (whatever you can afford) to:

   Canadians for Mercury Relief
   Suite 1812, 191 University Avenue
   Toronto, Ontario, Canada M5H 3M7
   (415) 410-6314; FAX (0-50 876-4203
   E-mail: communications@talkinternational.com

APPENDIX B

Physicians Knowledgeable About the Treatment of Dental-Filling Mercury Toxicity

New York

Warren Levin, M.D.
Comprehensive Medical
 Services
18 E 58th Street
New York, NY 10022
(212) 838-9100
FAX (212) 838-9903

Alfred Zamm, M.D.,
FACA, FACP
(914) 338-7766
111 Maiden Lane
Kingston, NY 12401-4597

Connecticut

Warren Levin, M.D.
31 Bailey Avenue
Ridgefield, CT 06877
(203) 894-8370

Florida

Joya Shoen, M.D.
341 N. Maitland Avenue
Orland, FL
(407) 644-2729

BLOOD SENSITIVITY TESTS

Walter J. (Jeff) Clifford, M.S.
(719) 550-0008, FAX 0009
P.O. Box 17597
Colorado Springs, CO 80935

Huggins Diagnostic Center
5080 List Drive at Centennial
Colorado Springs, CO 80919
(719) 548-1600
(800) 331-2303

INSTITUTIONAL REVIEW BOARD STUDY

In 1994, the Great Lakes Medical Association agreed to sponsor an Institutitional Review Board Study of mercury detoxification with DMPS, designed by Paula Bickle, Ph.D. and Dieter Klinghardt, M.D. To date, there are 92 participating physicians around the U.S.

For information concerning this study or for the name of a participating physician near you, contact:

Paula Bickle, Ph.D.
Cascade Health Group, Inc.
9310 Southeast Stark St.
Portland, Oregon 97216
(503) 256-9666
(306) 253-4445
Fax (503) 256-0053

APPENDIX C

General Reading List

There are not many titles on mercury toxicity published for the general reader, and even fewer written for physicians or scientists. As the public becomes more aware of this problem, undoubtedly this information gap will be filled. The few titles listed below constitute everything that is available in Fall 1996.

Many of these books cannot be found in bookstores or health food stores and must be ordered directly from the publisher. Publishing information such as address and price are included where available.

Fasciano, G.S. *Are Your Silver Dental Fillings Killing You?* This book contains a great deal of valuable information and scientific research.

Huggins, Hal A., DDS. *It's All in Your Head: Diseases Caused by Silver-Mercury Fillings.* Garden City Park, New York, 1993. Avery Publishing Company, $10.95. This highly readable and fascinating book from Avery Press is an excellent introduction to the subject of amalgam toxicity, with personal insights into Dr. Huggins' career.

Huggins, Hal A., D.D.S. *Proper Amalgam Removal*. Colorado Springs Life Sciences Press, (800) 331-2303. A step-by-step manual for removing mercury amalgam fillings and for following Huggins' detoxification regime.

Queen, Sam and Betty A. *The IV-C Mercury Tox Program (A Guide for the Patient)*. The Queens have reached the conclusion that intravenous vitamin C is the easiest and best way to detoxify if you are suffering from mercury poisoning. They have published an excellent three-part collection: a guide for the patient, a guide for the physician, and a hard-cover volume which gives all the scientific background for mercury amalgam filling removal and intravenous vitamin C detoxification.

Taylor, Joyal, D.D.S. *The Complete Guide to Mercury Toxicity from Dental Fillings*. $14.95. This is one of the most comprehensive books on dental amalgam and its removal, including photographs of correct masking of the patient. It can be ordered from Dr. Taylor's office, The Environmental Dental Association, 9974 Scripps Ranch Boulevard, Suite 36 San Diego, California 92131 Tel. (619) 586-1208; Fax (619) 693-0724.

Warren, Tom. *Beating Alzheimer's: A Step Towards Unlocking The Mysteries of Brain Diseases*. Garden City Park, New York: Avery Publishing Group, 1991. $12.95 in paper. This surprising book tells how the author, assisted by his pharmacist wife, decided to fight back against a diagnosis of Alzheimer's Disease and discovered that a brain allergy to his many mercury amalgam dental fillings was the source of his illness. Contains convincing illustrations—a "before" CAT scan of Warren's brain showing a concavity in the frontal lobe which is typical of Alzheimer's, and an "after" CAT scan of his brain returned to a normal shape.

Warren also adds very helpful lists of resources for further information. He has recently begun publishing his own newsletter for people concerned about mercury toxicity and Alzheimer's.

Ziff, Michael, D.D.S., and Sam Ziff. *The Missing Link? A Persuasive New Look At Heart Disease as It Relates To Mercury. Florida:* 1991. Bio-Probe, Inc., P.O. Box 608010, Orlando, 32860-8010. An extremely interesting book. Ziff, a heart disease victim himself before having his own amalgam fillings replaced, cites a number of scientific studies showing that mercury absorption can create abnormalities in nerve transmission to the heart and can cause the walls of the veins and arteries to contract, resulting in higher blood pressure.

Ziff, Sam. *Silver Dental Fillings. The Toxic Time Bomb* New Mexico: 1984. Aurora Press, P.O. Box 573, Santa Fe, 87504. $12.50. An extremely useful book containing a great deal of research-based information in a simplified format. The Ziffs' research knowledge is wide-ranging.

Ziff, Sam, Michael F. Ziff, D.D.S., and Mats Hanson, Ph.D., *"Dental Mercury Detox,"* June 1995: Bio-Probe, $3.95. Orlando, Florida: P.O. Box 608010, Orlando, Florida, 32860-8010. (407)

NEWSLETTERS

The Bio-Probe Newsletter is an exceptional source of information on the whole field of mercury toxicity. Published by Bio-Probe Inc., it combines easily accessible writing with the most up-to-date developments both scientifically and politically. Subscription price is $65 per year from: BIO-PROBE, Inc., P.O. Box 608010 5508 Edgewater Drive, Orland, FL 32860-8010, (800)-282-9670, or bpinfo@bioprobe.com.

The Holistic Dental Digest Plus. This unique and fascinating source of information about preventive dental health care, published by a leading preventive dentist for over 37 years, Dr. Jerome Mittelman and his wife, Beverly Mittelman. At $13.25, a year's subscription makes a great gift for friends and family—particularly familes with young kids. Write to: Holistic Dental Digest Plus, The Once Daily, Inc., 263 West End Avenue, #2A, New York, NY 10023.

BOOKS ON ASSOCIATED CONDITIONS

Barnes, Broda S., M.D., and Lawrence Galton. *HYPO-THYROIDISM: The Unsuspected Illness.* New York: Thomas Y. Crowell & Co., 1976.

William G. Crook, M.D. *THE YEAST CONNECTION. A Medical Breahthrough.* Professional Books, P.O. Box 3494, Jackson, Tennessee, 38301, 1983. $15.99.

Shirley S. Lorenazani, Ph.D. *CANDIDA: A Twentieth Century Disease.* Keats Publishing, Inc., 27 Pine Street (Box 876) New Canaan, CT 06840. $4.50

John Parks Trowbridge, M.D. and Morton Walker, D.P.M. *THE YEAST SYNDROME: How To Help Your Doctor Identify and Treat the Real Cause Of Your Yeast-Related Illness.* New York, Bantam Books, 1986. $4.95.

APPENDIX D

Following is a precis of the research findings to date on dental amalgam mercury and its interaction with the body. It was written by Murray Vimy, D.M.D, and Fritz L. Lorscheider, Ph.D. It is used here with their kind permission.

DENTAL AMALGAM MERCURY

M.J. Vimy and F.L. Lorscheider
Faculty of Medicine
Depts. of Medicine and Medical Physiology
University of Calgary
May 1993

BACKGROUND

Within the past decade several laboratories, including our own, have established in humans that mercury (Hg) vapor is continuously released from dental "silver" amalgam tooth fillings which contain 50% Hg by weight. (1-3) The release rate of this Hg is enhanced within 10 minutes after the occlusal (biting) surfaces of these amalgams are stimulated by chewing (1,2,4) or tooth brushing (3). Levels of Hg vapor in intra-oral air, both before and after chewing, correlate significantly with the number and type of amalgam fillings (2,4). With continuous chewing over a prolonged period (30 min.) the intra-oral air Hg vapor level remains elevated, and then slowly declines to basal levels 90 minutes after chewing ceases (4). A single amalgam filling will release 15 mg Hg/day into mouth air (5).

Our original estimate of Hg dose absorbed from dental

amalgams in a randomly selected group of human subjects was 20 mg Hg/day (4), and a compartmental model
for Hg body burden accumulation from 1-10,000 days
was proposed (6). Subsequent estimations of amalgam
Hg dose by other laboratories have varied from 1.2 - 27
ug Hg/day, with a current consensus of approximately
10 (range 3-17) ug absorbed/day (7,8), which is in contrast to a total of only 2.3 ug Hg (inorganic and organic
forms) being absorbed daily from food, water and air
(8,9). It is now believed that dental amalgams constitute the major source of Hg exposure in the general
population (8,10,11). This belief is supported by human
autopsy studies demonstrating significantly higher Hg
levels in brain and kidney of subjects with dental amalgams than in control subjects with no amalgams (12).
At least two-thirds of Hg excreted in urine is derived
from dental amalgam. (13).

Several important questions have been raised by
these clinical studies regarding the metabolic fate of
amalgam Hg vapor and its potential pathophysiological
consequences. To address these questions we employed
an experimental animal model in which sheep received
dental amalgam tooth fillings containing a radioactive
Hg tracer. Whole-body image scan and tissue analysis
revealed several possible uptake sites: oral tissues, jaw
bone. lung and gastrointestinal tract. Once absorbed,
the Hg rapidly localized in kidney and liver (14). Similar
studies in pregnant sheep indicate that both maternal
and fetal tissues begin to accumulate Hg within several
days following amalgam placement and this accumulation is progressive with time (15). Another study in
monkeys (whose dentition, diet, feeding regimen and
chewing pattern closely resemble those of humans),
likewise demonstrates high levels of Hg concentration
in kidney, intestinal tract and other tissues 4 weeks
after placement of amalgams (16). The primate kidney

continues to accumulate amalgam Hg for as long as 1 year after placement of such fillings (17) at levels comparable to those seen in sheep (18). Current investigations in sheep and primates are designed to resolve the possible pathophysiological significance of this phenomenon, and to evaluate parallel issues in humans. Preliminary reports indicate that kidney function in sheep (19) and intestine/gingivae bacterial populations in monkeys (20) are significantly compromised when these animals are exposed to dental amalgam Hg, and in humans both fertility and brain function may be altered (21).

These experimental findings are in marked contrast to opinions recently pronounced by spokesmen for the dental profession (22) and the American Dental Association. (23)

NOTES

1. Svare, C.W., Peterson, L.D., Reinhardt, J.W., Boyer, D.B., Frank, C.W., Gay, D.D., and Cox, R.D. (1981) The effects of dental amalgams on mercury levels in expired air. J. Dent. Res. 60, 1668-1671.
2. Vimy, M.J., and Lorscheider, F.L. (1985) Intra-oral air mercury released from dental amalgam. J. Dent. Res. 64, 1069-1071.
3. Patterson, J.E., Weissberg, B., and Dennison, P.J. (1985) Mercury in human breath from dental amalgam. Bull. Environ. Contam. Toxicol. 34, 459-468.
4. Vimy, M.J. and Lorscheider, F.L. (1985) Serial measurements of intra-oral air mercury: estimation of daily dose from dental amalgam. J. Dent. Res. 64, 1072-1075.
5. Gross, M.J. and Harrison, J.A. (1989) Some electro-

chemical features of the in vivo corrosion of dental amalgams. J. Appl. Electrochem, 19, 301-310.

6. Vimy, M.J. Luft, A.J., and Lorscheider, F.L. (1986) Estimation of mercury body burden from dental amalgam: Computer simulation of a metabolic compartmental model. J. Dent. Res. 65, 1415-1419.

7. Vimy, M.J., and Lorscheider, F.L. (1990) Dental amagam mercury daily dose estimated from intra-oral vapor measurements: A predictor of mercury accumulation in human tissues. J. Trace Elem. Exper. Med. 3, 111-123.

8. World Health Organization (1991) Environmental Health Criteria 118, Inorganic Mercury p. 36, WHO, Geneva.

9. Clarkson, T.W., Hursh, J.B., Sager, P.R., and Syversen, T.L.M. (1988) Mercury. In: *Biological Monitoring of Toxic Metals* (Clarkson, T.W., Friberg, L., Nordbert, G.F., and Sager, P.R., eds.) pp. 199-246. Plenum Press, New York.

10. Lorscheider, F.L. and Vimy, M.J. (1991) Mercury exposure from "silver" fillings. Lancet 337, 1103.

11. Clarkson, T.W., Friberg, L., Hursh, J.B., and Nylander, M. (1988) The prediction of intake of mercury vapor from amalgams. In: *Biological Monitoring of Toxic Metals* (Clarkson, T.W., Friber, L., Nordberg, G.F., and Sager, P.R., eds.) pp. 247-260, Plenum Press, New York.

12. Nylander, M., Friberg, L., and Lind, B. (1988) Mercury concentrations in the human brain and kidneys in relation to exposure from dental amalgam fillings. Swed. Dent. J. 11, 179-187.

13. Aposhian, H.V., Bruce, D.C., Alter, W., Dart, R.C., Hurlbut, K.M. and Aposhian, M.M. (1992) Urinary mercury after administration of DMPS: Correlation with dental amalgam score. FASEB J. 6, 2472-2476.

14. Hahn, L.J., Kloiber, R., Vimy, M.J., Takahashi, Y.,

and Lorscheider, F.L. (1989) Dental "silver" tooth fillings: A source of mercury exposure revealed by whole-body image scan and tissue analysis. FASEB J. 3, 2642-2646.

15. Vimy, M.J., Takahashi, Y., and Lorschedier, F.L. (1990) Maternal-fetal distribution of mercury (203-Hg) released from dental amalgam fillings. Am J. Physiol, 258, R939-R945.

16. Hahn, L.J., Kloiber, R., Lininger, R.W., Vimy, M.J., and Lorscheider, F.L. (1990) Whole-body imaging of the distribution of mercury released from dental fillings into monkey tissues. FASEB J. 4, 3256-3260.

17. Danscher, G., Hersted-Beindslev, and Rungby, J. (1990) Traces of mercury in organs from primates with amalgam fillings. Exp. Mol. Path. 52, 291-299.

18. Letters to the Editor (1991) Mercury released from dental fillings. FASEB J. 5, 236.

19. Boyd, N.D., Benediktsson, E. Vimy, M.J., and Lorscheider, F.L. (1990) Mercury from "silver" dental tooth fillings impairs sheep kidney function. Am. J. Physiol. 261. R1010-R1014.

20. Summers, A.O., Wireman, J., Vimy, M.J. and Lorscheider, F.L. (1990) Increased mercury resistance in monkey gingival and intestinal bacterial flora after placement of dental "silver" fillings. Am. Physiol Soc. Fall Meeting, Orlando, FL, Oct. 10, 1990. The Physiologist 33(4), A-116, 1990.

21. Society of Toxicology Annual Meeting (1992) Symposium: Toxicity assessment of mercury vapor from dental amalgams. The Toxcicologist 12, 6-7.

22. Letters to the Editor (1990) Dental silver tooth fillings. FASEB J.4, 1542-1543.

23. American Dental Association Divisions of Communication and Scientific Affairs (1990) When your patients ask about mercury in amalgam. JADA 120, 395-398.

APPENDIX E

Bibliography of Selected Scientific Research on the Health Effects of Mercury Accumulation from Dental Amalgam

A THE ABSORPTION OF MERCURY FROM DENTAL FILLINGS

Fritz L. Lorscheider, Ph.D. and Murray S. Vimy, DDS.
University of Calgary Medical School, Alberta, Canada.

Drs. Lorscheider and Vimy have shown definitively that mercury is continuously released from amalgam fillings, both as vapor and in microscopic particles, once the fillings are placed in the teeth. The mercury emitted from the fillings is transported to every part of the body via the air pathways, the digestive tract and the blood stream, and accumulates in tissues and organ systems.

1. *Dental Amalgam Mercury: Background.* (A summary of research results on dental amalgam mercury to date.) M. J. Vimy and F. L. Lorscheider, Faculty of Medicine

and Medical Physiuology, University of Calgary, Calgary, Alberta. May, 1993.

2. *Dental "Silver" tooth fillings: a source of mercury exposure revealed by whole-body image scan and tissue analysis.* By Leszek J. Hahn, Reinhard Kloiber, Murray J. Vimy, Yoshimi Takahashi, and Fritz L. Lorscheider. FASEB Journal, Vol. 3, Dec. 1989. pp. 2641-2646.

3. *Whole-body imaging of the distribution of mercury released from dental fillings into monkey tissues.* By Leszek J. Hahn, Reinhard Kloiber, Ronald W. Leininger, Murray J. Vimy, and Fritz L. Lorscheider. FASEB Journal, Vo. 4, Nov. 1990, pp.3256-3260.

4. *Mercury from dental "silver" tooth fillings impairs sheep kidney function.* By N.D. Boyd, H. Benediktsson, M.J. Vimy, D.E. Hooper, and F. L. Lorscheider. American Jounrnal of Physiology, No. 261, 1991, pp. R1010-1014.

5. *Maternal-fetal distribution of mercury (203HG) released from dental amalgam fillings.* By M.J. Vimy, Y. Takahashi, and F.L. Lorscheider. American Journal of Physiology, No. 258, 1990, pp. R939-945.

6. *SYMPOSIUM OVERVIEW: Toxicity Assessment of Mercury Vapor from Dental Amalgams.* By Peter L. Goering, W. Don Galloway, Thomas W. Clarkson, Fritz L. Lorscheider, Maths Berlin and Andrew S. Rowland. Journal of Fundamental and Applied Toxicology, vol. 19, 1992, pp. 319-329.

7. *Evaluation of the safety issue of mercury release from dental fillings,* Fritz L. Lorscheider and Murray J. Vimy. The FASEB Journal, Vol. 7, December 1993, 1432-1433.

8. *ADP-Ribosylation of Brain Neuronal Proteins Is Altered by In Vitro and In Vivo Exposure to Inorganic Mercury.* Pawel Palkiewicz, Henk Zwiers, and

Fritz L. Lorscheider. Journal of Neurochemistry,, Vol. 62, No. 5, 1994, pp. 2049-2052.

B. BASIC PHYSIOLOGICAL RESEARCH ON THE RELATIONSHIP OF BRAIN MERCURY ACCUMULATIONS FROM DENTAL AMALGAM MERCURY TO ALZHEIMER'S DISEASE

William R. Markesbery, M.D., William D. Ehmann, M.D., (and colleagues at the University of Kentucky's Sanders-Brown Center on Aging).

Drs. Markesbery's and Ehmann's experiments have shown that there are higher concentrations of mercury in the autopsied brains of patients who died of Alzheimer's than are present in the autopsied brains of patients who did not have Alzheimer's. In the Alzheimer's patients' brains, there are also lower concentrations of selenium and zinc, the two chief mineral antagonists of mercury. Markesbery and Ehmann have also demonstrated that there are higher concentrations of mercury in the brains of people who have more and larger amalgam dental fillings. Additional research is underway to link the presence of amalgam fillings more closely with the incidence of Alzheimer's.

9. *Trace element imbalances in isolated subcellular fractions of Alzheimer's disease brains.* By David Wenstrup, William D. Ehmann, and William R. Markesbery. Brain Research, No 533, 1990, pp. 125-130.

10. *Mercury imbalances in patients with neurodegenerative diseases.* W. D. Ehmann, E. J. Kasarskis, and W. R. Markesbery. (In Press)

C. MERCURY AS A CAUSE OF TUBULIN TANGLES SIMILAR TO THOSE FOUND IN ALZHEIMER'S DISEASE, AND THE DEVELOPMENT OF A NON-INVASIVE TEST FOR ALZHEIMER'S

Boyd E. Haley, Ph.D. (and colleagues.) Professor of Medical Chemistry and Biochemistry, Markey Cancer Center, University of Kentucky.

Dr. Haley has produced tubulin defects in laboratory cultures of brain tissue by adding a low concentration of mercury plus EDTA, a common food additive. Tubulin defects are thought to be the mechanism which produces the neurofibrillary tangles characteristic of Alsheimer's Disease. Haley has also identified the first biochemical marker for Alzheimer's, that is, an enzyme found in Alzheimer's patients cerebro-spinal fluid which is not found in normal persons and which could be used as one basis of diagnosis for the disease.

11. *HG2+ induces GTF-Tubulin interactions in rat brain similar to those observed in Alzheimer's Disease.* E. Duhr, C. Pendergrass, E. Kasarskis, J. Slevin & B. Haley. FASEB Journal, 1992. Abstract Dated December 3, 1991.

12. *HgEDTA Complex Inhibits GTP Interactions With The E-Site of Brain Beta-Tubulin.* Edward F. Duhr, James C. Pendergrass, John T. Slevin, and Boyd E. Haley. Toxicol. Appl. Pharmacol., 1993.

13. *DMSA acid partially restores tubulin intereactions to both Alzheimer's Diseased brains and to HG-EDTA treated control brains.* J.C. Pendergrass, E.F. Duhr, J.T. Slevin, and B. E. Haley. Experimental Biology 93 Abstract, dated November 17, 1992.

14. *Aberrant Guanosine Triphosphate-Beta-Tubulin Interaction in Alzheimer's Disease.* Sabiha Khatoon, Ph.D., Susan R. Campbell, B.S., Boyd E. Haley, Ph.D.

and John T. Slevin, M.D. Annals of Neurology, Vol. 26, No. 2, August 1989, pp. 210-215.

15. *Detection of glutamine synthetase in the cerebro-spinal fluid of Alzheimer diseased patients: A Potential diagnostic biochemical marker.* Debra Gunnersen and Boyd Haley. Proceedings of the National Academy of Science, Vol. 89, pp. 11949-11953, December 1992, Biochemistry.

D. MERCURY CHELATING AGENTS AND MERCURY ABSORPTION MEASUREMENT

H. Vasken Aposhian, Ph.D., University Department of Molecular and Cellular Biology, University of Arizona, Tucson, Arizona.

Dr. Aposhian has established, through carefully constructed experiments, that in people who have amalgam fillings two-thirds of the total body burden of mercury is the product of mercury absorption from amalgam dental fillings. He has also created a scoring system based upon the number of fillings and the number of surfaces on the fillings, quantifying the expression of the amount of dental amalgam in an individual's mouth. Finally, he has also been experimenting with chelating agents which might remove mercury accumulations from the body.

16. *Urinary mercury after administration of 2,3 di-mercaptopropane-1-sulfonic acid: correlation with dental amalgam score.* H. Vasken Aposhian, David C. Bruce, Wilfred Alter, Richard C. Dart, Katherine M. Hurlbut, and Mary M. Aposhian. The FASEB Journal, Vo. 6, April 1992, pp. 2472-2476.

17. *DMSA and DMPS—Water soluble antidotes for heavy metal poisoning.* H. Vasken Aposhian. American Review of Pharmacology and Toxicology, 1983, Vol. 23, 193-215.

18. *Determination and Metabolism of Dithiol Chelating Agents, XII. Metabolism and Pharmacokinetics of Sodium 2,3-Dimercaptopropane-2—Sulfonate in Humans.* Richard M. Maiorino, Richard C. Cart, Dean E. Carter and H. Vasken Aposhian. The Jourmal of Pharmacology and Experimental Therapeutics, 1991, Vol. 259 No. 2, pp. 808-814.

19. *MESO-2,3-DIMERCAPTOSUCCINIC ACID: Chemical, Pharmacological and Toxicological Properties of an Orally Effective Metal Chelating Agent.* H. Vasken Aposhian and Mary M. Aposhian.

E. MERCURY AND RENAL DISEASE

James S. Woods, Battelle Seattle Research Center and the University of Washington, Seattle, Washington, and colleagues.

Dr. Woods has been investigating how kidney tissue is damaged by the presence of maercury. He has also identified ways in which porphyrin relationships are disrupted by the presence of mercury, which could provide another type of marker to test for the presence of mercury in body tissues.

20. *Mercury-induced H2O2 production and lipid peroxidation in vitro in rat kidney mitochondria.* Bert-Ove Lind, Dennis M. Miller and James S. Woods. Biochemical Pharmacology, Vol. 42, 1991, Suppl. pp. S181-S187. Pergamon Press.

21. *Urinary Porphyrin Profiles as Biomarkers of Trace Metal Exposure and Toxicity: Studies on Urinary Prophyrin Excretion Patterns in Rats during Prolonged Exposure to Methyl Mercury.* James S. Woods, Miriam A. Bowers, and Holly A. Davis. Toxicology and Applied Pharmacology, Vol. 110, 1991, pp. 464-476.

22. *Enhancement of Gamma-Glutamylcysteine Syn-*

thetase mRNA in Rat Kidney by Methyl Mercury. James S. Woods, Holly A. Davis, and Robert P. Baer. Archives of Biochemistry and Biophysics, Vol. 296, No.1, July 1992, pp. 350-353.

23. *Quantitative Determination of Porphyrins in Rat and Human Urine and Evalution of Urinary Prophyrin Profiles during Mercury and Lead Exposures.* Miriam A. Bowers, Lauri J. Aicher, Holly A. Davis, and James S. Woods. The Journal of Laboratory and Clinical Medicine, St. Louis. Vol. 120, No. 2, pp. 272-281, August, 1992.

F. ANTIBIOTIC RESISTANCE

Anne O. Summers, Ph.D., Department of Molecular Biology and Microbiology, University of Georgia, Athens, Georgia

Dr. Summers has been engaged in research on gastrointestinal tract bacteria and their resistance to antibiotics, which is a serious and widespread medical problem. With the collaboration of Drs. Lorscheider and Vimy and Dr. Stuart Levy at Tufts University, she has demonstrated that bacterial resistance to antibiotics can be created by exposing g.i. tract bacteria to mercury, such as that absorbed into the g.i. tract through the presence of amalgam dental fillings in the mouth.

24. *"Silver" Dental Fillings Provoke An Increase in Mercury and Antibiotic Resistant Bacteria in the Mouth and Intestines of Primates.* Anne O. Summers, Murray Vimy and Fritz Lorscheider, The Alliance for the Prudent Use of Antibiotics (APUA) Newsletter, Fall 1991, Vol. 9, No. 3, pp. 4-5.

25. *Mercury Released from Dental "Silver" Fillings provokes an increase in Mercury- and Antibiotic-Resistant Bacteria in Oral and Intestinal Flora of Primates.*

Anne O. Summers, Joy Wireman, Murray J. Vimy, Fritz L. Lorscheider, Bonnie Marshall, Stuart B. Levy, Sam Bennett, and Lynne Billard. *Antimicrobial Agents and Chemotherapy*, April 1993, Vol. 37, No. 4, p. 825-834.

G. CLINICAL MEDICAL TREATMENT OF DENTAL-FILLING MERCURY TOXICITY

Alfred V. Zamm, M.D., FACA, FACP, 111 Maiden Lane, Kingston, New York 12401-4597

Reports on clinical treatment of a wide variety of illnesses linked to dental amalgam mercury toxicity by a dermatologist and allergy specialist.

26. *Candida Albicans Therapy: is there ever an end to it? Dental Mercury Removal: an effective adjunct.* Alfred V. Zamm, M.D., FACA, FACP. Journal of Orthomolecular Medicine, Vol. 1 No. 4, pp. 261-266.

27. *Dental Mercury: A Factor That Aggravates and Induces Xenobiotic Intolerance.* Alfred V. Zamm, M.D., FACA, FACP. Journal of Orthomolecular Medicine, Vo. 6 No. 2, Second Quarter 1991, pp. 67-77.

28. *Mercury and Dentistry: What the Sensitive Patient Should Know.* Alfred V. Zamm, M.D., FACA, FACP. The Mercury in Medicine and Dentistry Newsletter Quarterly, Vol. 1 No. 1, Autumn 1986, pp. 1-8.

29. *Removal of Dental Mercury: Often an Effective Treatment for the Very Sensitive Patient. Alfred V. Zamm, MD, FACA, FACP.* Journal of Orthomolecular Medicine, Vol. 5, No. 3, Third Quarter 1990, pp. 138-142.

H. RESEARCH ON THE IMPACT OF DENTAL MERCURY ON THE IMMUNE SYSTEM, BRAIN, AND NEUROLOGICAL SYSTEM.
David Eggleston, D.D.S.

30. *Effect of dental amalgam and nickel alloys on T-lymphocytes: preliminary report.* Eggleston, David W. DDS. Journal of prosthetic dentistry: May 1984, Vol 31, No. 5.

31. *Correlation of dental amalgam with mercury in brain tissue.* Eggleston David W. DDS, Magnus Nylander DDS, et al. J. Pros. Dent. 58:704-7, 1987

32. *Dental Amalgam: A Review of the Literature.* Eggleston, DW: Compend. Cont. Ed. Dent. Vol. X, No. 9.

APPENDIX F

News Clippings

Scientist Parallels Dental Amalgams and Lead Poisoning

by Tom Paulson
P-I Reporter (Seattle)

Despite safety reassurances from the dental profession and two federal panels, leading toxicologists said evidence still points to mercury in amalgam dental fillings as a potentially serious health threat.

A Food and Drug Administration official, speaking at a Seattle meeting of the Society of Toxicology, drew parallels between the evidence against lead poisoning 20 years ago and the evidence against mercury today. Lead has since been proven harmful to humans and removed from paint, pipes and many other materials.

New evidence indicates a need for more vigorous study of the possible risk posed by the release of mercury vapor from "silver" amalgam fillings, said Dr. Don Galloway, a scientist with the FDA's Center for Devices and Radiological Health in Rockville, Maryland.

Making an analogy to lead poisoning, he said the rule of thumb for safety in lead exposure used to be the point at which exposure caused obvious physical symptoms. But studies have since shown that chronic exposure to even low levels of lead, especially in children, can cause significant developmental and neurological damage.

"Lead was removed from paint in 1971," Galloway said. Mercury was removed from paint in 1991, he noted, asking the toxicology group meeting at the Washington State Convention and Trade Center to consider if there is a 20-year lag between understanding mercury toxicity compared with lead toxicity. About 3,000 toxicologists attended the meeting.

"There are some striking similarities in the history," he said.

Galloway was careful not to say the mercury vapor emitted by the amalgams (the fillings are made of a mercury and silver alloy, along with other metals) has been shown to be harmful. Based on evidence, Galloway does not intend to have his own amalgam fillings replaced, but said he would prefer his children receive alternatives when possible. Common alternatives are plastic composites or porcelain fillings.

Scientific panels, one sponsored by the FDA and another by the National Institutes of Health, have said there is no evidence of a health threat posed by amalgam fillings.

But another toxicologist at the meeting, one whose work likely prompted the creation of both federal panels, said the dental profession and the U.S. regulatory system are choosing to ignore the data.

"These were preordained conclusions (of safety)," said Dr. Fritz Lorscheider from the University of Calgary in Alberta.

Lorscheider and his colleague, Dr. Murray Vimy, were the latest to renew the flap over dental amalgams with the 1990 publication of a study that reported reduced kidney function in sheep fitted with the fillings. Featured on CBS' "60 Minutes," the study was attacked by dentists and others who noted that sheep chew much more than humans. Critics also noted the sheep received their 12 fillings at one time, which would be atypical in humans.

But at the Seattle conference, Lorscheider reported finding similar data in monkeys, which chew like humans, and other evidence indicating that the standard methods of measuring mercury exposure give inaccurately low readings.

Most studies of exposure to mercury have based their measurements on blood and urine concentrations, Lorscheider said. New studies indicate that much of the mercury is retained in tissue, especially in the kidneys and liver, he said.

"There is an impairment in kidney function in animal studies," Lorscheider said. He added that certain regions of the brain also appear to concentrate mercury.

If mercury-silver amalgams were to be proposed today as a new medical or dental device, he said the scientific evidence of potential risk would be enough to prevent them from ever reaching the market.

"Dental amalgam is a major source of mercury in the general population," Lorscheider said.

Other speakers at the panel on amalgams generally supported the contention that dental amalgams could pose a health risk.

But several in the audience, some of them dentists, questioned the validity of some of the research.

An epidemiological study by a researcher at the National Institutes of Environmental Safety and Health purported to show reduced fertility in dental assistants with high exposure to mercury. The scientist said other factors affecting fertility had not been ruled out.

◆

Germany Bans One Form of Silver/Mercury Dental Fillings!

On February 1, 1992, the German Ministry of Health declared a ban on one form of silver/mercury dental fillings. This action, to be effective March 1, 1992, has been taken on medical grounds because of adverse health effects in patients exposed to mercury released from amalgam fillings. Confirmation of this dramatic action was reported at the winter meeting of the International Academy of Oral Medicine and Toxicology (IAOMT), held in Orlando, Florida, February 1 & 2, 1992, by the president of the German chapter of the IAOMT.

The IAOMT program covered the recently published research findings of medical scientists demonstrating the harmful effects of mercury exposure from the dental filling. These findings include damage to the kidneys, placental passage of mercury to unborn babies, and increased resistance to various antibiotics, which has

become a very serious medical treatment problem. Additional research information was presented demonstrating probable relationship of mercury exposure to Alzheimer's disease and to cardiovascular disease.

An overview was also presented at the annual meeting of the Society of Toxicology held in Seattle, Washington February 23-27, 1992. At this meeting, world class toxicologists and scientists presented additional medical research on the subject of mercury exposure and its harmful effects. Research findings showed that pre-natal exposure to mercury vapor can cause learning deficits and behavioral problems. These affects are similar to those causing great medical concern about lead levels in children. The results of another study showed reduced fertility in dental assistants who are occupationally exposed to mercury vapor from amalgam. This study corroborates a recently

published study indicating harmful effects of mercury on male fertility.

The German announcement together with the scientific data presented from prestigious medical sources contradicts the pervasive public pronouncements by the American Dental Association, the Food and Drug Administration and the National Institute of Dental Research that silver/mercury dental fillings are harmless to patients. Further statements claiming that amalgam dental fillings are safe are contrary to the scientific evidence, and clearly not in the best interests of the public health.

Further information, confirmation of all statements, and selected interviews may be arranged by calling Dr. Michael F. Ziff, Executive Director of the IAOMT at 407-293-0136, or writing IAOMT.

◆

Townsend Letter for Doctors June 1992

MERCURY NEWS
SAN JOSE, CA

Wednesday, December 15, 1993

3B

California News

Dentists to post warnings of mercury in fillings

BY MIRANDA EWELL
Mercury News Staff Writer

SAN FRANCISCO — Marking a major break in a decadelong controversy, some California patients visiting their dentists will soon notice a sign warning, them that the mercury in their dental fillings can cause birth defects.

On Tuesday, one of the nation's largest manufacturers of mercury amalgam dental fillings agreed to put Proposition 65 warnings on its packages and provide signs for California dentists to display in their offices. The agreement, which came as part of a settlement with an Oakland-based environmental law group, signals the first time in the United States that such warnings will be provided to consumers.

"A major part of the (dental) industry has agreed to break the wall of silence and put in people's hands the information that mercury in fillings causes birth defects," said James Wheaton, president of the Environmental Law Foundation.

"There is no reason to panic," Wheaton added. "Your teeth are not killing you, but you have the right to this information and the people who should be most cautious are those who are pregnant or who are planning to have a child in the next decade."

The signs will read: "WARNING: This office uses amalgam filling materials which contain and expose you to mercury, a chemical known to cause birth defects and other reproductive harm. Please consult your dentist for more information."

Wheaton said he did not know how many California dentists are supplied by Jeneric/Pentron Inc. of Wallingford, Conn., the company that agreed to the

WARNING

This office uses amalgam filling materials which contain and expose you to mercury, a chemical known to cause birth defects and other reproductive harm. Please consult your dentist for more information.

A maker of mercury dental fillings will provide warnings on packages and signs in some dental offices.

birth defect warnings. But the environmental group hopes that other major manufacturers of the mercury amalgam dental fillings and three dozen distributors will follow Jeneric's lead, he said.

The Connecticut company declined to comment on the agreement. The Environmental Law Foundation sued Jeneric in San Francisco Superior Court under the provisions of Proposition 66, passed by voters in 1986 to provide information to consumers on chemicals that can cause birth defects and reproductive problems. In the settlement, Jeneric agreed to provide the warnings within 46 days to dentists it supplies.

Dental amalgam, the "silver" filling that typically consists of 40 percent to 54 percent elemental mercury, is widely used.

"There is evidence that women who work in dental clinics and regularly handle mercury amalgam have observable reproductive problems," said Dr. William Pease, a research toxicologist at the University of California, Berkeley School of Public Health.

Epidemiological studies show that female dental workers experience altered menstrual cycles and increased rates of spontaneous abortion, Pease said. Studies are inconclusive at this time regarding the effects of mercury amalgam dental fillings on patients, he said. But the toxicologist noted that minute amounts of mercury vapor can escape from the amalgam when cavities are filled or during vigorous chewing.

"There is no question women who work in an environment where mercury is present need to be warned," Pease said. "Whether patients are at risk from the dental amalgam is still a question."

No safety thresholds have been established for exposure to mercury, he said.

A growing number of dentists are concerned about the mercury issue, said James Rota, a Los Angeles dentist.

Rota, who has practiced for 34 years and used to teach about mercury fillings at the University of California, Los Angeles, said he has not used mercury fillings for 17 years.

"The information has been frightening," said Rota, who called mercury fillings an "occupational hazard" for dentists. "Personally, I don't think mercury belongs in the mouth at all".

Rota said he believed mercury fillings were linked to problems with the immune system. He himself got so sick with symptoms that mimicked those of chronic fatigue syndrome that he was unable to work.

Eventually, Rota said, he had his own mercury fillings removed, although he did not recommend that for everyone. Removal must be done carefully, with adequate safeguards, he said.

Internationale Akademie für Oral-Medicine und Toxicologie Europa e.V.
I.A.O.M.T.-Europa e.V.

Shadow Strase 28
40212 Düsseldorf
Deutschland.
Tel 0211-133533
Fax 0211-133555
Steuernummer 1331242888
23-12-93

"Out for Amalgam"

Degussa stops production.

Degussa AG has, with immediate effect, stopped the production of the controversial tooth filling material Amalgam.

A spokesman for the firm in Hanau - until now the largest manufacturer of mercury products in Germany - stated that amalgam use was declining throughout the world. Moreover, the production site was to be moved from Pforzeim to Hanau to dedicate a great increase in the development of an alternative filling material. The spokesman stated that the cessation of production had no connection to the Wesseling based patient group, IGZ, that had made a complaint to the Frankfurt Prosecutor. The IGZ lodged a complaint over half a year ago against Degussa claiming severe injury to the body by the use of amalgam.

The likely real reason is that next year a new law of the European Union will/may (under discussion but Germany has said it is likely to agree to it) come into action. This law states that if a a party thinks he has been damaged by a product, he no longer has to prove damage, the manufacturer must prove that it could not happen. This is a reversal of the present situation, the onus of proof being transferred. You can imagine the consequences of such a law. So can Degussa.

Yours

Graeme Hall, B.D.S., F.I.A.O.M.T. President I.A.O.M.T. Europa e.V.

Aus für Amalgam.

Degussa stellt Produktion ein

Die Degussa AG stellt „ab sofort" die Produktion des umstrittenen Zahnfüllstoffes Amalgam ein. Wie ein Sprecher des Unternehmens – bislang bundesweit größter Hersteller des quecksilberhaltigen Werkstoffs – in Hanau mitteilte, geht der Amalgamverbrauch „weltweit zurück". Außerdem werde die Produktionsstätte von Pforzheim nach Hanau verlagert, wo man sich „verstärkt der Entwicklung alternativer Füllstoffe" widmen wolle. Der Unternehmenssprecher bestritt, daß die Produktionseinstellung mit einem Ermittlungsverfahren in Zusammenhang stehe, das unter anderem die „Interessengemeinschaft Zahngeschädigter" (IGZ) mit Sitz in Wesseling bei Köln gegen die AG bei der Frankfurter Staatsanwaltschaft ins Rollen gebracht hatte. Die IGZ hatte vor anderthalb Jahren wegen des Verdachts vorsätzlicher schwerer Körperverletzung durch den Einsatz von Amalgam Strafanzeige erstattet.

NOTES

Preface
1. See Appendix F for a translation of the newspaper article announcing this decision; also, interview with De Gussa official in the BBC Panorama TV program, "The Poison In Your Mouth."
2. The American Medical Association, Resolution introduced by Michigan Delegation, 12/92.
3. *San Jose Mercury News*, December 15, 1993. See Appendix F.
4. *Bio-Probe Newsletter*, Vol. 9 Issue 2, March 1993, pp. 7/8.
5. W. H. Tolhurst vs Johnson & Johnson Consumer Products, Inc.; Engelhard Corp; ABE Dental, Inc.; The American Dental Association, et al. In *the Superior Court of the State of California, In and For the County of Santa Clara. Case No. 718228*

Chapter 1
They Aren't Really Silver
6. Environmental Protection Agency, quoted in presentation by Marcia Basciano, D.D.S., at Annual Meeting of IAOMT, San Diego, Cal. October 1994.
7. Personal communication from Dr. Fritz Lorscheider and Dr. Murray Vimy.
8. Sam Ziff, *THE TOXIC TIME-BOMB: Can the Mercury*

In Your Dental Fillings Poison You? Aurora Press,
Box 573, Santa Fe, N.Mex., 87504. p. 9f.

9. There have been a number of incidents in the second
half of the 20th Century in which human beings have
been inadvertently poisoned by mercury that acciden-
tally made its way into foodstuffs.

The most famous incident was the contamination
over many years of the waters of Minamata Bay in
Japan by the Chisso Corporation, whose Minamata
plant secretly dumped mercury-containing effluent into
the sea on a continuing basis for almost 40 years (1932
to 1971). Bacteria in the seawater changed the effluent's elemental mercury into the more poisonous
methyl mercury; algae consumed the bacteria and were
in turn eaten by fish, which were caught and eaten by
the townsfolk of this traditional fishing village.

Over a period of years the villagers of Minamata
experienced first mild symptoms of a mysterious illness, then more advanced symptoms and finally terrifying deformities. Everyone was affected: newborns,
children, adults. Although the Chisso Corporation
eventually made some reparations, it never acknowledged the extent of the damage done nor the number
of persons injured. The illness persisted long after
dumping had ceased; by 1982, 1,773 people had been
formally declared victims of the disease; 459 of these
had actually died; and 5,000 cases remained to be
processed, at the painfully slow rate of 50 per month.

The villagers' terrible odyssey was documented by
American photographer W. Eugene Smith and his
wife Aileen M.Smith, who took up residence in the
town so as to record more faithfully the villagers' daily
life. The resulting photographs and text were published in **MINAMATA: The Story of the Poisoning of
a City and of the People Who Chose to Bear The
Burden of Courage.** (Holt, Rinehart and Winston,

1975.) Smith paid dearly for his altruism; he was attacked by thugs hired by Chisso and brutally beaten. Although he lived for some years after the beating, eventually he died of those injuries.

Minamata was and remains a stunning and profoundly moving testament to the extreme qualities of good and evil which human beings can express. We are accustomed to seeing photographs of such extraordinary deformities in the wake of war or pestilence. Instead, they are products of corporate carelessness and greed—the unwillingness of a few individuals to confront the consequences of their actions for the whole community. Minamata has also provided us, tragically, with a vast textbook of the wide range of illnesses and dysfunctions produced by mercury poisoning.

Another great mass of information on the effects of mercury poisoning has been furnished by a series of incidents halfway around the world from Minamata. The middle of this century saw a tragic succession of mercury poisoning incidents in Iraq, in 1956, 1960, 1970, and 1972, which were a result of mercury's entry into the food chain in a very different way. American seed wheat sent to Iraq for planting was treated by Iraqi officials with a mercury-containing fungicide to prevent mildew (a common problem for seed grain that must be stored for long periods of time.) In four separate incidents, villagers who did not know that the wheat had been treated with mercury and could not read the labels on the bags, ground this seed wheat and used it for food, with appalling results.

The last of these incidents is said to have been the most catastrophic. 6,530 persons were admitted to hospitals, and 459 persons died. Since then, Sweden has proposed and adopted a protocol avoiding the use of mercury-containing fungicides internationally, and has been followed in this by a number of other nations. Meanwhile scientists have mined and distilled the aftereffects of the poisoning among hundreds of villagers.

For fuller descriptions of the Iraqi incidents, see Chronic Mercury Toxicity: New Hope Against An Endemic Disease. Doctor's Guide for Lifestyle Counseling, Volume 1. H.L. Queen. Queen & Company Health Communications, Colorado Springs, Colo., 1988, pp. 17-19 and passim.
10. BIO-PROBE Newsletter, March 1993, Vol. 9, Issue 2, Page 1.
11. Ibid, p. 7.
12. Ibid, p. 7.
13. David Eggleston, D.D.S. Effect of dental amalgam and nickel alloys on T-lymphocytes: preliminary report. Journal of Prosthetic Dentistry: May 1984, Vol 31, No. 5.
Chapter 2
What We Know About Mercury
14.
Elemental mercury (Hg^0) and Mercury Vapor

Elemental mercury has a core of 120 neutrons and 80 protons, with a surrounding cloud of 80 electrons. Two of these electrons are unstable: they can be lost to other compounds. When elemental mercury is in contact with bacteria (in the water or soil) or with enzymes (in the human body), these organisms act like biochemical muggers: their enzymes or oxidizing agents grab two mercury electrons from any mercury atom they encounter and run off with the stolen electrons. This creates a second form of mercury, Hg^{2+}, which has two "holes" in its electron ring where the missing electrons once were. ($2+$ means that it can acquire two new electrons,)

These "holes" in the electron ring of $Hg2+$ are what enables mercury to do so much damage in the human body. They transform mercury into a marauder in its turn. Once the two electrons have been stolen, the mercury atom is voracious to get them back. Like a crime victim obsessed with vengeance, its only objective is to refill the two holes in its rim. So the mugged molecule becomes a mugger: mercury then combines with any other substance it encounters in the body that has available electrons it can seize—such as chloride or sulfur atoms, for example, both quite common in the human body. When combined with these two elements it is known as "inorganic mercury."

A mercury molecule that has attached itself to an electron fron another element <u>has combined chemically with that element</u>. In doing so, it creates a new compound with characteristics and qualities that are different from those of either of the individual elements. Sometimes this difference intensifies an element's worst qualities. When the highwayman form of mercury, Hg^{2+} combines with carbon and chloride, it creates **Organic Mercury, ($CH_3Hg^+Cl^-$)**, also called "methyl mercury chloride" or "methyl mercury" for short. Methyl mercury is acknowledged to be the most poisonous form of mercury in existence.

I am indebted for most of this information to Dr. Anne Summers, whose skill in teaching the fundamentals of chemistry applies just as effectively to adult writers as it does to graduate students in biology.

15. The Committee To Coordinate Environmental Health and Related Programs, Public Health Service, U.S. Government. Dental Amalgam: A Scientific Review and Recommended Public Health Service Strategy for Research, Education and Regulation. Final Report of the Subcommittee on Risk Management. January 1993.

16. International Symposium on "Status Quo Perspectives of Amalgam and Other Dental Materials," *Europaeum*, European Academy Otzenhausen, Germany, April 19-May 1, 1994.

17. Personal communication from Fritz Lorscheider, Ph.D.
18. Leszek, 1989.
19. World Health Organization, l992.

Chapter 3
The Lorscheider-Vimy Experiments
20. Svare, C.W., Peterson, L.D., Reinhardt, J.W., Boyer, D.B., Frank, C.W., Gay, D.D., and Cox, R.D. (1981) The effects of dental amalgams on mercury levels in expired air. *J. Dent. Res.* 60, 1668-1671.
21. Vimy, M.J., and Lorscheider, F.L. (1985) Intra-oral air mercury released from dental amalgam. *J. Dent. Res.* 64, 1069-1071.
22. *The Federation of American Societies of Experimental Biology*
23. Scientific measures are made in the metric system throughout the world. Measurements for mercury content are given in nanograms, micrograms, milligrams, and grams. A kilogram (2.205 pound) contains a thousand grams; a gram contains a thousand milligrams; a milligram contains a thousand micrograms; and a microgram contains a thousand nanograms. A nanogram is one billionth of a gram; a microgram is one millionth of a gram; a milligram is one thousandth of a gram; a gram is one thousandth of a kilogram; and a kilogram is equal to 2.205 pounds.
24. Hahn, L.J., Kloiber, R., Vimy, M.J., Takahashi, Y., and Lorscheider, F.L. (1989) Dental "silver" tooth fillings: A source of mercury exposure revealed by whole-body image scan and tissue analysis. *FASEB J. 3*, 2642-2646.
25. Hahn, L.J., Kloiber, R., Lininger, R.W., Vimy, M.J., and Lorscheider, F.L. (1990) Whole-body imaging of the distribution of mercury released from dental fillings into monkey tissues. *FASEB J. 4*, 3256-3260.

26. Boyd, N.D., Benediktsson, E. Vimy, M.J., and Lorscheider, F.L. (1990) Mercury from "silver" dental tooth fillings impairs sheep kidney function. Am. J. Physiol. 261. R1010-R1014.

27. Ibid.

28. For a more recent update of related research, see Lorscheider et al, FASEB Journal 9:504-508, 1995.

Chapter 4
The Link Between Mercury and Alzheimer's Disease

29. Wenstrup, David, Ehmann, William D., and Markesbery, William R. Trace element imbalances in isolated subcellular fractions of Alzheimer's disease brains. Brain Research, No 533,1990, pp. 125-130.

30. Thompson, C., Markesbery, W., Ehmann, W. Mao, Y., and Vance, D. (1988). Regional brain trace-element studies in Alzheimer's disease. Neurotoxicology. 9, 1-7.

31. 25. Eggleston David W., DDS, Magnus Nylander DDS, et al. Correlation of dental amalgam with mercury in brain tissue. J. Pros. Dent. 58:704-7,1987.

32. Aposhian, H. Vasken, Bruce, David C., Alter, Wilfred, Dart, Richard C., Hurlbut, Katherine M., and Aposhian, Mary M. Urinary mercury after administration of 2,3 dimercaptopropane-1-sulfonic acid: correlation with dental amalgam score. The *FASEB Journal*, Vol. 6, April 1992, pp. 2472-2476.

33. Duhr, Edward F., Pendergrass, James C., Slevin, John T., and Haley, Boyd E. HgEDTA Complex Inhibits GTP Interactions With The E-Site of Brain BetaTubulin. Toxicol. Appl. Pharmacol., 1993.

34. Pendergrass, James C., Haley, Boyd E., Lorscheider, Fritz L., and Vimy, Murray D. Neurotoxicology/5 (4): 955, 1994

35. Gunnersen, Debra and Haley, Boyd E. Detection of glutamine synthetase in the cerebrospinal fluid of Alzheimer diseased patients: A Potential diagnostic

biochemical marker. *Proceedings of the National Academy of Science,* Vol. 89, pp. 11949-11953, December 1992, Biochemistry.

Chapter 5
The Immune   System, Antibiotic Resistance, and Other Mercury-linked Syndromes

36. David Eggleston, D.D.S. Effect of dental amalgam and nickel alloys on T-lymphocytes: preliminary report. *Journal of Prosthetic Dentistry*: May 1984, Vol 31, No. 5.
37. Eggleston, ibid.
38. David Eggleston, D.D.S. Effect of dental amalgam and nickel alloys on T-lymphocytes: preliminary report. *Journal of Prosthetic Dentistry*: May 1984, Vol 31, No. 5.

Citations from article by Dr. David Eggleston:

3. Aiuti, F. and Pandolfi, F. The role of T-lymphocytes in the pathogenesis of primary immunodeficiencies, *Thymus* 4:257, 82.
8. Stingl, G., Garza, L.A., Czarnecki, N. and Wolf, K.T. T-Cell abnormalities in atopic dermatitis patients: imbalances of T-cell subpopulations and impaired generation of Con-A induced suppressor cells. J. Invest. *Dermatol.* 76:468, 91.
10. Chateroud, L., and Bach, M.A. Abnormalities of T-cell subsets in glomerulonephritis and systemic lupus erythematosus. *Kidney Int.* 20-267, 1981.
11. Frazer, I. H. and MacKay, I. R. T-lymphocyte subpopulations defined by two sets of monoclonal antibodies in chronic active hepatits and systemic lupus erythematosus. Clin. Exp. Immunol. 50:107, 1982.
12. Cagnoli, L, Tabbachi, P, Pasquali, S, Cenci, M, Sasdelli, M., and Zucchelii, P. T-cell subset altera-

tions in idiopathic glomerulonephritis. *Clin. Exp. Immunol.* 50:70, 1982.

13. Traugou, U., Reinherz, E.L., and Raine, C.S. Multiple sclerosis: Distribution of T-cell subsets within active chronic lesions. *Science* 219:308, 1983.

14. Oleske, J., Minnefor, A., Cooper, Jr., R., Thomas, K., del Cruz, A., Abdieh, H., Gerrero, I., Joshi, V.V., and Desposite, F. Immune Deficiency syndrome in children. *J. Am. Med. Assoc.* 249:2345, 1983.

15. Rubenstein, A., Sticklick, M., Gupta, A., Bernstein, L., Klein, N. Rubinstein, E., Spiglann, I., Fruchter, L., Liman, N., Le, H., and Hollander, M. Acquired Immunodeficiency with reversed T4/T8 ratios in infants born to promiscuous and drug-addicted mothers. *J. Am. Med. Assoc.* 249:2350. 1983.

16. Sonnabend, J., Witkin, S.S., and Purtilo, D.T. Acquired immunodeficiency syndrome, opportunistic infections, and malignancies in male homosexuals. *J. Am Med Assoc.* 249:2370, 1983.

19. Butler, M., Atherton, D., and Levinsky, R.J. Quantitative and functional deficit of suppressor T-cells in children with atopic eczema. *Clin Exp Immunol.* 50-02, 1982.

20. Reinherz, E.L, Weiner, H.L., Hauser, S. L., Cohen, J.A., Distaso, J.A., and Scholossman, S.F. Loss of Suppressor T cells in active multiple sclerosis. *N. Engl. J. Med.* 303:125, 1980.

21. Morimoto, C., Reinherz, E.L., Schlossman, S.F., Schur, P.H., Mills, J.A. and Steinberg, , A.D.: Alterations in immunoregulatory T cell subsets in active systemic lupus erythematosus. *J. Clin. Invest.* 66:171, 1980.

22. Kohler, P.F., and Vaughn, J.: The autoimmune diseases. *J. Am. Med. Assoc.* 248-2446, 1982.

81. Newman, S., Chamberlain, R.T., and Nunez, L.J.: Nickel solubility from nickel chromium dental casting alloys. *J. Biomed. Mater. Res.* 15:615, 1981

83. Fisher, J.R., Roseblum, G.A., and Thomson, B.D. Asthma induced by nickel. *J. Am.Med. Assoc.* 248:1065, 1982.
123. Reinherz, G.L., Geha, R., Wohl, M.E., Morimoto, C., Rosen, F.S., and Schlossman, S.F. Immunodeficiency associated with loss of T4+ inducer T-cell function. *N.Engl. J. Med.* 304:811, 1981.

39. Hultman, Per, Johannson, Uno, Turley, Shannon J., Lindh, Ulf, Enerstrom, Sverker, and Pollard, K. Michael. Adverse immunological effects and autoimmunity induced by dental amalgam and alloy in mice. *The FASEB Journal*, Vol. 8, No. 14, Nov. 1994, pp. 1183-1190.
40. Summers, Anne O., Wireman, Joy, Vimy, Murray J., Lorscheider, Fritz L., Marshall, Bonnie, Levy, Stuart B., Bennett, Sam, and Billard, Lynne. Mercury Released from Dental "Silver" Fillings provokes an increase in Mercury- and Antibioti-Resistant Bacteria in Oral and Intestinal Flora of Primates. *American Society for Microbiology: Antimicrobial Agents and Chemotherapy*, April 1993, Vol. 37, No. 4, p. 825-834.

Chapter 6
MedicalImplicationsofMercuryToxicity:Alfred Zamm, M.D., F.A.C.P.

41. From personal interview with Alfred A. Zamm, M.D., F.A.C.A., F.A.C.P. See also Mercury and Dentistry: What the Sensitive Patient Should Know. Alfred V. Zamm, M.D., FACA, FACP. *The Mercury in Medicine and Dentistry Newsletter Quarterly*, Vol. 1 No. 1, Autumn 1986, pp. 1-8.

Chapter 7
The Huggins Diagnostic Center:
Hal A. Huggins, D.D.S.

42. Huggins, Hal A., D.D.S., M.S. *It's All In Your Head: The Link Between Mercury Amalgams and Illness.* New York: Avery Publishing Group, 1993, p. xi.
43. Ibid.

Chapter 8
How Can I Tell If I'm Mercury Toxic?

44. Based on an estimate by Sugita, M. in *The Biological Half-Time of Heavy Metals. The Existence of a Third and Slowest Component. International Archives of Occupational Health,* Vol. 41, p. 25, 1978.
45. Arvidson, B. (1987) Retrograde axonal transport of mercury. *Exp. Neurology,* 98, 198-203.
46. Chang, L. W., and Hartman, H.A., Blood-Brain Barrier Dysfunction in Experimental Mercury Intoxication, *Acta Neuropthology,* Vol. 21, pages 179-184, 1972.
47. Yoshino, Y., Mozai T., and Nakao K., *Journal of Neurochemistry,* Vol. 13, pages 1223-1230, 1966.
48. Hunter et al, Poisoning by Methylmercury Compounds. *Quarterly Journal of Medicine,* Vol. 33, pp. 193-206, 1941. See also Garman, R. H., Weiss, B., and Evans, H.L., Alkylmercurial Encephalopathy in the Monkey (Samiri Scieureus and Macaca Arctoides) A Histopathologic and Autoradiographic Study. *Acta Neuropathology* (Berlin) Vol. 32, Issue 1, pp. 61-74, 1975.
49. Huggins, Hal A., D.D.S., *IT'S ALL IN YOUR HEAD: Diseases Caused by Silver-Mercury Fillings.* Colorado Springs, Colorado: Life Sciences Press, 1989.
50. Amin Zaki et al, Methylmercury Poisoning in Iraqui Children, Clinical Observations Over 2 Years, British

Medical Journal, Vol. 1, Page 613, 1978. Cited in Sam Ziff, *Silver Dental Fillings: The Toxic Time Bomb*, p.86.

51. Ziff, Michael F. D.D. S, and Sam Ziff, *The Missing Link? A Persuasive New Look At Heart Disease As It Relates To Mercury.* 1991, Bio-Probe, Inc., Orlando, Florida.

52. Amin-Zaki L. et al. Prenatal methylmercury poisoning. *Am. J. Dis. Child*, 133:172-177, 1979.

53. Ziff, Sam, *SILVER DENTAL FILLINGS: The Toxic Time Bomb*, p. 95.

54. Smith, W. Eugene, and Smith, Aileen M. *MINAMATA: The Story of the Poisoning of a City, and of the People Who Chose To Carry The Burden Of Courage. An Alskog-Sensorium Book.* New York: Holt, Rinehart and Winston, 1975.

55. Tejning, S. Mercury Levels in Blood Corpuscles and in Plasma in "Normal" Mothers and Their New-Born Children. *Report 68 02 Z from Dept. of Occupational Medicine*, University Hospital, Lund, Sweden, Lung Stencils, 1968.

56. Vimy, M.J., Takahashi, Y., and Lorschedier, F.L. (1990) Maternal-fetal distribution of mercury (203-Hg) released from dental amalgam fillings. *Am J. Physiol*, 258, R939-R945.

57. Reuhl, K.R. and Chang, L.W., Neurotoxicology, Vol.I, pp. 21-55, 1979; Clarkson T.W., et al, Dose-Response Relationships for Adult Pre-natal Exposures to Methyl Mercury, . In Measurement of Risks, G.G. and H.D. Mialle, editors, Plenum, New York, 1981; and Marsh, D.O. et al, Fetal Methylmercury Poisoning: Clinical and Toxicological Data on 29 Cases. Annals of Neurology, Vol. 7, pp. 348-453, 1980. Cited in Ziff, Sam, *SILVER DENTAL FILLINGS: The Toxic Time Bomb,* p. 105.

58. Mercury burden of human fetal and infant tissues, Gustave Drachts et al, Institut for Reichsmedizin,

Munich. Eur. J. *Pediatrics*, 1994, Vol. 153 pp. 607-610.

59. See Lorsheider and Vimy studies already cited and Ziff book *SILVER DENTAL FILLINGS: The Toxic Time Bomb* already cited for specific results and for lists of scientific studies.
60. Goldman, M and Blackburn, P. 4*The effect of mercuric chloride on thyroid function in the rat.* Toxicol. Appl. Pharmacol. 48:49-55. 1979.
61. Synthroid, a popular artificial thyroid medication, is a different form—T3—that has to be turned into T4 by the body. Thus it takes a greater energy expenditure for the body to make use of it.
62. For a fuller description see Broda S. Barnes, M.D.: *Hypothyroidism*.
63. Ziff, Sam. *SILVER DENTAL FILLINGS: The Toxic Time Bomb*, p. 75.
64. Huggins, Hal A., D.D.S. *IT'S ALL IN YOUR HEAD: Diseases caused by Silver-Mercury Fillings.* Colorado Springs: Life Sciences Press, pp. 47-59.
65. Ziff, Sam. Op cit., pp. 96-101.
66. Ibid, pp. 99-100.
67. Ibid, p. 100.
68. Fiskesjo, G. The Effect of Two Organic Mercury Compounds on Human Leukocytes in Vitro. *Hereditas*, Vol. 64, pp.142-146, 1970.
69. Hultman, Per, Johannson, Uno, Turley, Shannon J., Lindh, Ulf, Enerstrom, Sverker, and Pollard, K. Michael. Adverse immunological effects and autoimmunity induced by dental amalgam and alloy in mice. *The FASEB Journal*, Vol. 8, No. 14, Nov. 1994, pp. 1183-1190.

General Index

Acrodynia, 108
ADD (Attention Deficit
  Disorder), 72
Allergies, 8
Alzheimer's Disease,
  53–64
American Medical
  Association (AMA),3
Anemia, 20
Apoe, 60-61
Arsenic, 8
Arthritis, 119
Asthma, 66

B-Complex Vitamins,
  22
Behavior, 109
Blood, 106
Brain, 8, 63, 64,106,110
Breasts, 98
Bronchial Tubes, 66
Bruxism, 110

Cadmium, 8
Calomel, 109
Candida, 100
Chang and Hartman, 91
Composites, 120
Crohn's Disease, 100
Depression, 10
Dermatitis, 13, 110
Detoxification, *83–87*
DMPS, 56, 125, 126, 129
DMSA, 126, 129

Ears, 66
Eczema, 110
EDTA,
Electrogalvinism, 24
Endocrine glands, 8
Environmental Law
  Foundation, 3
Esophagus, 70
Eyesight, 65–66

Fatigue,
Frequent urination, 71

Gastrointestinal Tract,
    8n, 10
Gingivitis, 10, 63
Glandular System, 73
Goiter, 20
Gum tissues, 63

Hatter's Syndrome, 109
Heart, 8,94-95
Heme, 55–56
Hemoglobin, 107
HIV, 119
Hormones, 105

Immune System, 75
Intestinal Tract, 70–71
Irritable Bowel
    Syndrome, 100

Kidneys, 8, 71, 106

Leukocytes, 106,
Liver, 8
Lungs, 66
Lupus, 119
Lymphocytes, 106

McGraw-Hill Encyclo-
pedia of Science and
    Technology, 20

Memory Problems, 107
Mercury (HG),
    Inorganic mercury,
        23 ff.
    Symptoms of acute
        exposure, 20–21
    Symptoms of chronic
        exposure, 20–21
Minamata, 104
Miscarriage, 104
Monkeys, 31–42
MS, 119
Muscles, 8, 20–21

OSHA standards for
    dental mercury
    disposal, 21

Pituitary, 104, 106
Pleva, Jaro, 92
Porphyrins, 55–56
Psoriasis, 110

Reproductive Tract, 104

Selenium, 128
Sheep, 31–42
SIDS, 105
Sinuses, 63
Skin diseases, 108
Stomach, 70
Sulfhydryls, 13
Sweden, 4

Throat, 66

Thyroid, 21, 73, 106
 Hypothyroidism, 106
Tongue, 64

Vagus nerve, 64
Van Nostrand's Scientific Encyclopedia, 20

Vitamin B1, Thiamin--
 Vitamin B6, 127
Vitamin C, 18, 127

Zinc, 90

Index of
Proper Names

ADA (American Dental Association), xvii, xviii, 23, 26

AMA (American Medical Association), 3

Aposian, H. Vasken, Ph.D., *44–45*, 48

Aposian, Mary, Ph.D., *44–45*, 48

Barnes, Broda S. M.D. 146

BBC, xvii

BioProbe, 139

Breiner, Mark, D.D.S., 101

Carolynska Institute, 4

Carroll, Louis, 19

Clifford, Walter, J., 116-118, 142

Crawcour Brothers, 26

Crook, William, G., M.D. 146

DAMS, 139-40

Echevarria, Diana, Ph.D.,

Eggleston, David, D.D.S., 14, 23, 30, 55-56, 65-67, 135

Ehmann, William, Ph.D., 53–64

Encyclopedia Americana, 20

Encyclopedia Britannica, 20

Encyclopedia Law Foundation, xvi

EPA (Environmental Protection Agency), 23, 28, 38

Fasciano, Guy, 143

FASEB (Federated Association of Societies of Experimental Biology), 42, 70

FDA (Food and Drug
Agency), 12

Goodman and Gilman's
Pharmacological
Basis of Theraputics,
22,
Grismaijer, Soma, 99

Haley, Boyd, Ph.D., 14
16, 31, 53-64
Hamlet, 20
Hankla, John, D.D.S.,
136
Hanson, Matts, Ph.D.,
8, 145
Hindin, Howard, D.D.S.,
136
Huggins, Hal A., D.D.S.,
30, 81-84, 93, 108,
135-136, 142-144

IAOMT, 136
Iraq, 103

King, Wayne, D.D.S.,
136

Levin, Warren, M.D.
141
Levy, Stuart, Ph.D.,
70
Lichtenberg, Hanrik,
D.D.S., 12

Lorenzani, Shirley S.,
146
Lorscheider, Fritz L.,
Ph.D., 5,6, 14, 31,
147-151, 153-155

Marshall, Bonnie, 70
Masi, James V., 24-25
Markesbery, William,
M.D., 14, 53-64
McGraw Hill Encyclo-
pedia of Science, 21
Minamata, 103

OSHA, 13

Queen, Sam and Betty,
144

Pleva, Jaro, 65
Pinto, Olympio, D.D.S.,
30, 136
Pollard, K. Michael, 67-
68

Schoen, Joya, M.D., 141
Shakespeare, William,
20
Siblerud, Robert L. ,
O.D., M.S., 11
Singer, Sydney Ross, 99
Sorrin, Bruce, D.D.S.,
136
Steiner, Alan, D.D.S.,
136

Summers, Anne O.,
    Ph.D., 31, 68-74,
    104

Taylor, Joyal D., D.D.S.,
    135, 144
Trowbridge, John Parks
    M.D., 146
Tufts University, 70

University of Calgary
    Medical School, 5
University of Georgia,
    31
University of Southern
    California, 23

Van Nostrand's Scienti-
    fic Encyclopedia, 21

Vimy, Murray, D.D.S.,
    5-6, 14, 30-31, 34-52
    70, 106, 147-51, 153-155

Ward, Frank, D.D.S.,
    136
Warren, Tom, 144
World Health Organiza-
    tion, 23, 34
Woods, James, Ph.D.,
    55–56

Zamm, Alfred V., M.D.,
    FACP,
    12, 58-60, 101, 128, 141
Ziff, Michael, D.D.S.,
    8-11, 75-79 103, 145
Ziff, Sam, 11, 103, 145